STEROIDS

**Recent Titles in
Health and Medical Issues Today**

STEROIDS

Aharon W. Zorea

Health and Medical Issues Today

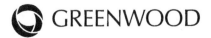 GREENWOOD

AN IMPRINT OF ABC-CLIO, LLC
Santa Barbara, California • Denver, Colorado • Oxford, England

Library of Congress Cataloging-in-Publication Data

Zorea, Aharon W., author.
  [Steroids (Zorea)]
  Steroids / Aharon W. Zorea.
     p. ; cm. — (Health and medical issues today)
  Includes bibliographical references and index.
  ISBN 978-1-4408-0299-7 (hardcopy : alk. paper) — ISBN 978-1-4408-0300-0 (ebook)
  I. Title.   II. Series: Health and medical issues today.
  [DNLM: 1. Steroids—adverse effects.   2. Steroids—therapeutic use.
3. Anabolic Agents. QU 95]
  RM297.S74
  615.3'6—dc23   2014000217

ISBN: 978-1-4408-0299-7
EISBN: 978-1-4408-0300-0

18 17 16 15 14   1 2 3 4 5

This book is also available on the World Wide Web as an eBook.
Visit www.abc-clio.com for details.

Greenwood
An Imprint of ABC-CLIO, LLC

ABC-CLIO, LLC
130 Cremona Drive, P.O. Box 1911
Santa Barbara, California 93116-1911

This book is printed on acid-free paper ∞

Manufactured in the United States of America

CONTENTS

SERIES FOREWORD

Every day, the public is bombarded with information on developments in medicine and health care. Whether it is on the latest techniques in treatment or research or on concerns over public health threats, this information directly affects the lives of people more than almost any other issue. Although there are many sources for understanding these topics—from websites and blogs to newspapers and magazines—students and ordinary citizens often need one resource that makes sense of the complex health and medical issues affecting their daily lives.

The *Health and Medical Issues Today* series provides just such a one-stop resource for obtaining a solid overview of the most controversial areas of health care in the 21st century. Each volume addresses one topic and provides a balanced summary of what is known. These volumes provide an excellent first step for students and laypeople interested in understanding how health care works in our society today.

Each volume is broken into several sections to provide readers and researchers with easy access to the information they need:

- Section I provides overview chapters on background information—including chapters on such areas as the historical, scientific, medical, social, and legal issues involved—that a citizen needs to intelligently understand the topic.
- Section II provides capsule examinations of the most heated contemporary issues and debates and analyzes in a balanced manner the viewpoints held by various advocates in the debates.
- Section III provides a selection of reference material, such as annotated primary source documents, a time line of important events, and

a directory of organizations that serve as the best next step in learning about the topic at hand.

The *Health and Medical Issues Today* series strives to provide readers
with all the information needed to begin making sense of some of the most
important debates going on in the world today. The series includes volumes on such topics as stem-cell research, obesity, gene therapy, alternative medicine, organ transplantation, mental health, and more.

INTRODUCTION

Steroid use is a multidimensional issue for health and medicine, and one deserving comprehensive discussion. They are biological chemicals, and when introduced to the human body, every steroid will cause a reaction—some of them are intended and desirable, while other reactions are unintended and possibly harmful. Through the careful manipulation of steroids, doctors are able to sidestep the internal feedback mechanisms that operate within the body to treat a wide variety of diseases and other ailments. But there is always a cost because, no matter how localized the intended application of the steroid hormone, it can never be limited to just one function or one location. When these same drugs are used for nontherapeutic purposes, then the costs can be much greater, and the question of appropriate usage is often removed from the hands of scientists and placed into the hands of policymakers, philosophers, and fundamentally falls to each individual. Therein lies the source of debate.

Steroids are not easily classified according to their structure, their function, or their eventual use. They include hormone and nonhormone variants and are used for therapeutic and nontherapeutic purposes. Among athletes, the questions of inappropriate use of anabolic steroids mostly involve fairness, player safety, and integrity of the game. Yet, these issues are often confused by the numerous therapeutic uses for the same kinds of steroids outside of sports. Among patients, the question of appropriate use requires a thoughtful balance between short-term benefits and potential long-term costs. Catabolic steroids are prescribed for ailments ranging from allergy suppression and anemia to life-threatening diseases, including degenerative arthritis, blood disorders, memory loss, and certain cancers. Often, the discoveries made for therapeutic treatments can also be adapted for sport-related performance enhancement. In this way, the pressure of adapting to constant innovation is shared by both catabolic and anabolic steroids.

Considerable material for public debate can be found in issues related to both catabolic and anabolic steroids—whether it involves economic-political tensions related to regulating cholesterol or the bioethical debates over the cost-benefit analysis of the therapeutic use of corticosteroids, or the sociopolitical conflict over the use of anabolic androgens for performance enhancement, or the philosophical dilemma of trying to evade old age. For both catabolic and anabolic steroids, these questions lead to some common issues: (1) Where should the locus of authority be for deciding (or regulating) these answers; (2) To what degree should public government be involved in educating (or compelling) agreement; and (3) At what point must scientific innovation admit the limitations of moral and ethical safeguards?

These and other issues related to steroid use can be arranged into more manageable policy questions according to the sectors of society that they most affect. Individuals must make decisions about their acceptable risk. State governments must create prohibitions when individual decisions impact the larger society. Private associations establish a cultural tone that greatly influences both the individual decision maker and state intervention. Throughout the book, we examine each sector individually, and then collectively. The following questions will emerge as common themes:

- **Individual Health:** What role should the individual play in determining their personal health choices, especially those that balance short-term relief against long-term disability? What guidelines should they use when making those determinations and who should be involved in setting those guidelines? How do age, gender, and mental development impact the available options and the individual's ability to choose them? Are there limits to individual decision making?
- **State/Public Health:** To what extent should governmental agencies be involved in regulating appropriate usage for the sake of protecting public health? When do the preferences of the government interfere with the individual freedom to make their own health decisions? What responsibilities does private industry have in protecting consumer health and is that responsibility best determined by the government or by the consumer? What measures should government take in treating abuse when it becomes apparent? When does government regulation go too far?
- **Private Associations and Sports Industry:** At what point do the regulations of sport associations interfere, overlap, or transcend

governmental authority or individual prerogative? What responsibility does the sports industry play in promoting suitable expectation of public health? How do sport associations measure fairness in an age when the natural diversity of individual ability may be offset by scientific and technological aids? Are there some non-sports-related associations that have a greater justification for enhancing personal performance?

This book is arranged so that these questions are presented systematically and topically. Section I (Chapters One, Two, and Three) provides an overview of the technical, historical, and cultural issues related to steroid use. The first chapter defines the biochemical nature of both kinds of steroids, while the second and third chapters provide historical backgrounds for catabolic and anabolic steroids respectively. Section II (Chapters Four, Five, and Six) applies these issues to existing policy decisions that confront individuals, lawmakers, and various private associations. Chapter Four discusses the factors that influence medical decision-making process for individuals, while Chapter Five considers the extent to which the government helps to predetermine the available options that individuals will face. The final chapter examines the degree to which private organizations can influence public debate. Last, Section III (Appendixes A, B, and C) supplies a collection of primary source materials that may serve as useful starting points for further discussion of both catabolic and anabolic steroids.

Continual research and development into a variety of steroid-based solutions for life-altering ailments necessitates constant vigilance among individual consumers, among the public, and among regulatory bodies of professional and amateur athletics organizations. The purpose of this book is to provide the reader with a comprehensive understanding of steroids both as a medical and as a cultural issue.

SECTION I

Overview and Historical Background

CHAPTER 1

Basics of Biochemistry and Steroids

Steroids form a very broad umbrella of organic chemicals that human life—indeed, all life—depend upon every day. It is impossible to avoid using steroids internally, and it is increasingly more difficult to avoid one or more of their variants externally. Steroids are used for a wide variety of therapeutic purposes as well as for enhancing physical performance. Popular culture generally associates steroids only with those anabolic androgen-based drugs used and abused by famous athletes that fill the newspapers with scandal. In fact, steroids are used by millions of people every day to treat or regulate certain changes in their body—some by need and others by desire. Two of the most widely prescribed drugs in the world, asthma inhalers and oral contraceptives, are based on the synthetic versions of cortisol and progesterone steroids, neither of which have any noticeable impact of enhancing physical strength or endurance.

Before discussing the many medical, political, and social issues that the research and development of various synthetic steroids has inspired, it is first necessary to better understand what steroids are, how they function, and to what end they are most often administered. This will necessarily include a little biology, chemistry, pharmacology, and a great deal of endocrinology. After this, the various policy issues arising from both the therapeutic and performance-enhancement uses of steroids should become most apparent. Mostly, they involve questions about appropriate use and the management of risk.

STEROIDS AND HORMONES IN HUMAN PHYSIOLOGY

Steroids are a form of hormone, which is an organic compound that helps to regulate the chemical reactions in the human body. There are several broad categories of steroids, and each category includes hundreds of related varieties, including more than 600 anabolic androgens alone. Thousands of different chemical compounds are forged and broken to produce an untold number of reactions that occur every moment, unseen within the human system. To fully understand the role and importance of steroids within this myriad complex of interrelated systems, it may be necessary to step back and start with an overview of human biology.

The Various Systems in the Body

The human body is a living machine that is fueled when we eat and drink and breathe. Part of that fuel is converted into energy needed to sustain all functions, while another part is used to build and maintain existing tissues (such as bone, muscles, and hair). Whatever remains after this conversion process is then excreted out of the body. Taken as a whole, the broad process of biochemical reactions needed to sustain all life is called **metabolism**. Those metabolic operations that help to break down materials are called **catabolism**, and those operations that build up and sustain existing tissues are called **anabolism**. Most of our human organs each play a crucial role in facilitating these anabolic and catabolic conversions.

When we eat and drink, the material passes through our digestive system (stomach and intestines), where it is broken down into the component proteins. At the same time, when we breathe in and out, oxygen is exchanged with carbon dioxide and other gasses through our respiratory system (lungs). The circulatory system includes a vast network of veins and blood vessels that carries both proteins and gasses to each organ throughout the body, and it is driven by the pulmonary system (heart). The physical shape and structure of our bodies is defined and supported by our muscular and skeletal systems, which provides mobility and contributes some metabolic functions. The nervous system uses an even more complex network (brain, spinal cord, and nerves) to transmit information through electrochemical waves that coordinates the various systems into a complimentary whole. Some of these instructions are consciously directed, such as the movement of our muscles to control our hands or legs, but most of the instructions that pass along the peripheral nervous system are automatic and occur below our conscious control. This is what allows us to think of other things through the day rather than having to consciously remind ourselves to breath, to sweat, or to regulate our heartbeats.

The **endocrine system** also serves to coordinate the functions of the various organs. Rather than using electrochemical waves directed from the brain through the neural networks, the endocrine system sends out various chemical compounds through the blood stream to regulate most of our metabolic functions. Through a combination of hormones and enzymes, the endocrine system sustains a vast network of interdependent chemical reactions that operate at the cellular level to tell each organ when to start, stop, or vary their rate of functions. **Hormones** are specialized chemical compounds that affect the permeability of cell membranes, govern the rate of chemical reactions (including cascading chains of reactions), activate or inhibit enzyme systems, and influence the functions of genes at the chromosomal level.

The Role of Steroid Hormones

The specific process of hormonal interaction is mostly chemical. A hormone is released from an organ or one of the adrenal glands (or occasionally from other tissues) and enters into the blood stream, where it passes by cell tissues throughout the body. Steroid hormones are fat soluble and **hydrophobic**—which means they do not like water but they do like other fats. Just like oil and water, hormones remain distinct from water-based systems and only operate inside other fat-soluble tissues. Blood is mostly water, while human cells are mostly fats. While in the bloodstream, steroid hormones are enwrapped by unique proteins that bind to it and protect it from the water-based blood plasma, thereby allowing the steroid hormone to pass through unchanged. Each protein wrapper is unique to certain kinds of steroids, and they lead the hormone to the appropriate cells. Different kinds of cells attract and contain receptors for specific kinds of hormones.

When the hormone passes by an appropriate cell, it is drawn into it through the cellular membrane (because it, too, is hydrophobic). In the process, the steroid loses its protein wrapper and passes into the cytoplasm where it connects with a unique receptor protein that is waiting for it. Some steroid types, estrogen for example, will find their receptor proteins on the cell membrane as well as in the cytoplasm, and that means the reactions occur more quickly. Others may find their receptor protein in the cell nucleus itself, which means the reaction processes are a bit slower. Regardless of where the receptors are located, once the steroid binds with its receptor protein, the entire mechanism moves into the nucleus where it interacts directly with the chromosomal enhancers that effectively turn on or turn off the functions of particular genes.

Genes are made of DNA strands that determine the particular characteristics of the organism, and they are responsible for the synthesis of certain

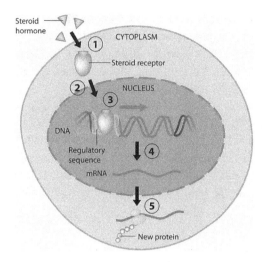

Diagram of a steroid hormone response. (Alila07/Dreamstime.com)

proteins. When the steroid and its accompanying receptor enter the nucleus, they create a copy of the relevant strand on the DNA chain, which is responsible for activating (or inhibiting) whatever operation that cell was programmed to undertake. This copying process is called **transcription**, and it results in a messenger of sorts (called messenger RNA—or **mRNA** for short) that then interacts with **ribosomes**, which is an acid molecule that "reads" the mRNA and links appropriate amino acids together to create the correct protein. The entire process is called **translation**, and it is sometimes referred to as the expression of a gene's function.

For our purposes, it is important to note that steroids are like the key used to unlock certain proteins, including the synthesis of other steroids, which in turn triggers a cascade of chemical interactions that produce a necessary result in one or more of the body's systems. The presence or absence of a particular hormone plays a critical role in regulating the growth and function of tissues at the cellular level. Hormones are responsible for growth, physical healing, and sexual reproduction. They can also have a significant impact on our mood and reaction to pain. Hormones are the primary medium for metabolic function.

The Perfect Balance

Like any chemical reaction performed in laboratory setting, the interaction between hormones and their protein receptors occur without any conscious choice on the part of the hormone or the protein receptor. In the most basic terms, a signal is received, a hormone is released, and a reaction follows. There are certain chemical-based **feedback loops** built into the endocrine system that help to guard against overproduction or underproduction of certain hormones. The delicate balance of chemical interactions is automatically governed through various glands, especially the pituitary gland located at the base of the brain, which monitors the rate of hormone production. The endocrine system relies on this broader feedback cycle to control the production of hormones and enzymes in order to maintain a harmonious balance called **homeostasis**. Nevertheless, if certain hormones come in contact with their receptors, then the chemical reaction will occur regardless of whether it adheres to the natural protective thresholds set by the endocrine system. Chemical reactions occur when the two reagents are placed in contact—reactions do not depend on the intelligent determination of benefit or harm. This opens the possibility that individuals might try to manipulate their hormone systems in ways that were not possible through their naturally occurring conditions.

Our hormonal balance greatly influences our physical appearance, our internal functioning, and our general health and well-being. Height, size, weight, and even age and gender characteristics are largely based on hormonal interactions. External influences such as environment, diet, and exercise also add to the mix, but the general balance is largely defined by parameters that are unique to our particular physiological profile. Under ideal circumstances, these parameters function in harmony, resulting in good general health. In some situations, though, one or more of these interrelated systems may begin to work independently—producing too many hormones or too few for the individual profile—resulting in one of many health-related diseases.

Hormonal Manipulation

Our modern pharmaceutical industry is largely the result of researchers seeking therapeutic solutions for medical disorders through customized drug combinations that seek to add to those processes where there are hormonal deficiencies and disrupt those processes where there are hormonal excesses. Unfortunately, the metabolic system is so interconnected that it is very difficult to address the deficiency in one area without creating an excess in another. That is why almost every drug has unwanted side effects. For the most part, doctors strive to find solutions that guarantee the greatest benefit to the patient with the least amount of harmful side effects—and they have been generally successful. Over the last 50 years, the public has welcomed these medical breakthroughs and our current society relies heavily on chemical supplements to maintain public health.

At the same time, however, as the pharmaceutical industry begins to understand the biochemical interactions operating within our bodies, new pressures arise to stimulate very specific hormonal reactions that can enhance physical performance in an otherwise healthy system. If we can isolate the hormones that lead to stronger muscles, then the professional athletes may be tempted to enhance their natural abilities with artificial supplements. Every supplement, whether taken for therapeutic or for performance purposes, has potentially harmful side effects. It is this last point that is most relevant for the discussion of both the use and abuse of steroids and other hormones.

OVERVIEW OF STEROID CHEMISTRY

In terms of human biology, steroids are part of a complex system of hormones and enzymes that interact together to sustain human life. Yet, from a chemical perspective, steroids belong to a much larger family of molecules that can be found in virtually all life-forms—plant and animal. This universality makes steroids extremely important to biochemists because once they understand the relationship between similar forms, then they can use non-human sources to create new artificial compounds for human use. Though part of a living system, steroids are necessary and essential to chemical compounds that react in predictable ways. The more scientists understand the basic chemical properties of steroids, the more likely they are to replicate, or very closely imitate those compounds that trigger specific metabolic reactions. This pursuit is the basis of most modern pharmacological research.

The Chemical Structure

A steroid is an organic, fat-soluble compound comprising 17 carbon atoms arranged in three cyclohexane (six-membered) rings and one cyclopentane (five-membered) ring connected side by side. This basic structure, called **gonane**, is common to all steroids. For the sake of clarity, chemists

Gonane

(Courtesy of Brandon Fetterly)

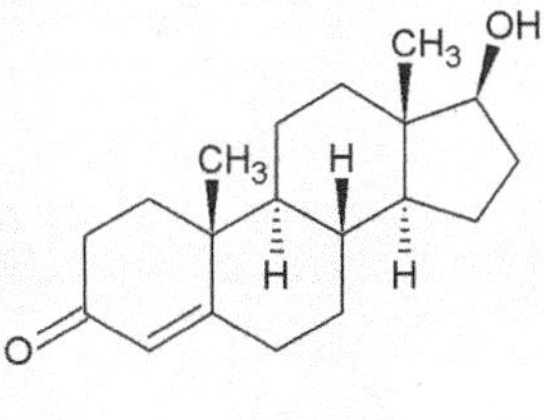

Testosterone

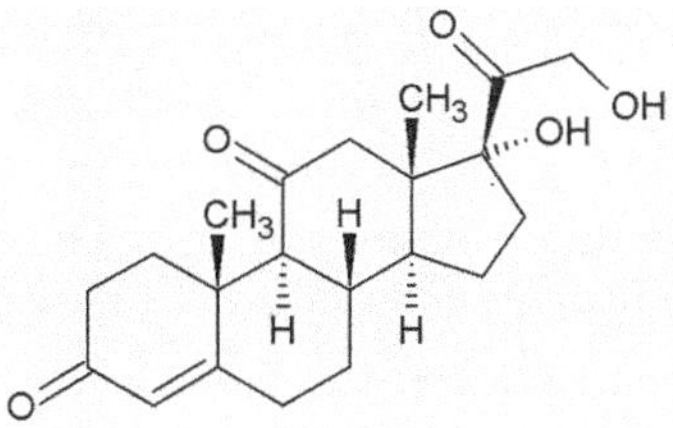

Cortisone

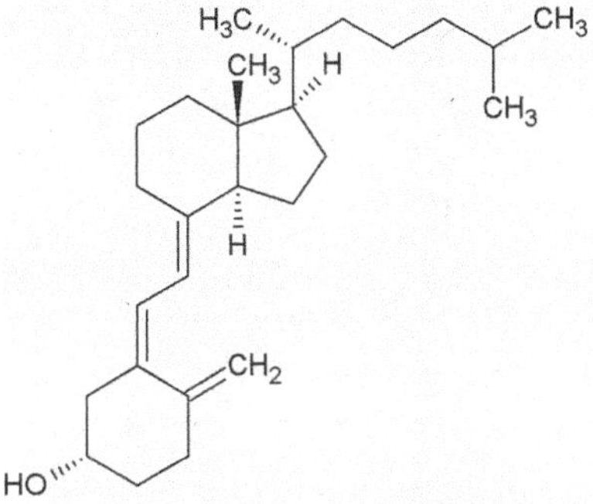

Vitamin D

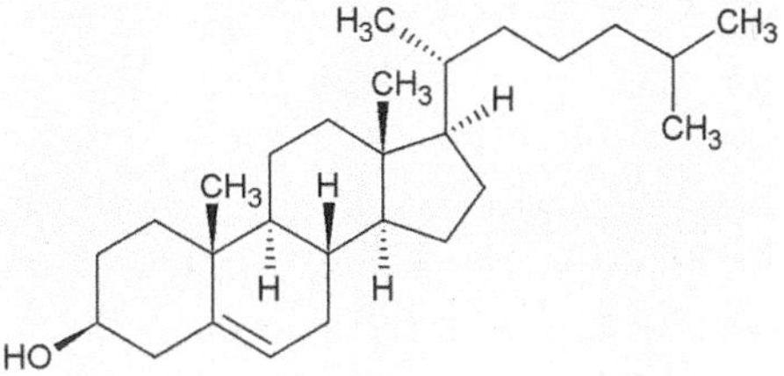

Cholesterol

(Courtesy of Brandon Fetterly)

do not label the carbon or connected hydrogen atoms when they draw pictures of their molecular structure, but we can assume that there is one carbon atom at each joint where the sides of the rings connect. The carbon atoms are numbered from 1 to 17 and the rings are labeled A, B, C, and D. This limited structure is, however, incomplete because there are three points (at carbon numbers 5, 14, and 17) where the carbon atoms are most likely to bond to another molecule. The added **moiety** (which is a piece of another molecule) is called a **substituent** because it *substitutes* for the hydrogen atom on the gonane, and the addition of one or more moieties is what really distinguishes one steroid from another. The unique molecular structure allows for thousands of compound combinations, all of which still adhere to the basic steroidal shape. Most of the natural steroid molecules form bonds at the seventh carbon atom, which adds a tail to the basic gonane structure. Some of the most common naturally occurring steroids, including testosterone, cortisone, cholesterol, and progesterone, all have stereoisomer bonds on the 17th carbon atom.

Natural Metabolism (In Vivo Synthesis)

The differences between one steroid molecule and another may be very slight, but each shape corresponds to a particular steroid receptor protein in a cell's cytoplasm, resulting in unique chemical reactions. Each molecule will produce a unique effect, sometimes quite distinct from another. At the same time, the similarity between steroidal molecules also helps to explain the interrelationship between one hormone and another. For example, cholesterol and vitamin D differ only in the broken bonds on the B ring and an added CH_3 substituent along the tail. Yet, they each serve much different purposes in the body. Vitamin D is used for the metabolism of calcium, which helps to strengthen bone tissues, while cholesterol is a sort of mother steroid from which most other hormones are derived; in its unchanged form, it is used largely in the construction of cell walls, which in human physiology are referred to as **cell membranes**. The close connection between the two molecules is important because the transition from cholesterol to vitamin D can occur relatively easily by passing the material under ultraviolet light.

Part of the metabolic processes at the cellular level occurs when tissues synthesize one hormone into another. When this occurs within a living organism, the process is called **in vivo** synthesis. For example, the liver, intestines, skin, and other organs can combine acids, enzymes, and proteins (acetate, mevalonic acid, squalene, and lanosterol) to synthesize cholesterol. In turn, cholesterol is metabolized into progesterone by the liver and kidneys. It is also metabolized into testosterone by the gonads. Progesterone can, in turn, be metabolized into corticosteroids by the liver and kidneys, while testosterone can be metabolized into estrogen by the ovaries. Each steroid molecule retains the same basic structure with three cyclohexane rings and one cyclopentane ring and differs only by the type and location of their substituent. Yet, in one instance, the steroid may be used to build up tissues (such as anabolic testosterone), while another may be used to break down tissues (such as the catabolic corticosteroids).

In Vitro Synthesis

On paper, the transition from one hormone molecule to another is as simple as moving one atom or isotope molecule from one location to another. In actual practice, the transition can be quite difficult to implement—only vitamin D can be synthesized under the relatively simple process of adding energy through ultraviolet light. Most other molecules require numerous intervening steps to take it from one form to another. Chemists try to discover and identify those steps in what they call the **synthesis pathway**. Artificial synthesis is difficult because chemists cannot pick out single atoms and arrange them as they like—even with our most sophisticated equipment, individual atoms are far too small to manipulate mechanically.

Instead, chemists rely on their knowledge of the properties of known molecules to use their unique bonds to attract or sever particular atoms and moieties from other molecules. The resulting chemical reactions may lead to seemingly disconnected changes, but each reaction can potentially bring about the building blocks for another reaction that eventually produces the desired transformation.

The process of **in vitro** synthesis of steroid compounds (when chemists try to replicate synthesis in a laboratory) is often quite complicated, and usually involves a great deal of trial and error. We can visualize the difficulty of chemical manipulation by imagining a Rubik's cube. Transforming a completed cube into a new "O" design seems relatively simple. It begins with a starting position where all six sides are solid colors and ends at a new position where the centers of each side seem to have been moved around. Both the starting and end results are very similar to each other, with only a single square on each side being moved. In fact, the process required dozens of steps in between the first and last position, during which time the manipulation seems to throw the cube into a confusion of colors until the final result is reached. Similarly, chemists who want to create an artificial steroid synthesis are often forced to undertake dozens of reactions with a variety of chemical compounds to force the transition of one substituent from one position on the steroid molecule to another.

Fortunately, research groups record and publish their findings, and over time certain predictable reactions can be discerned and isolated through experimentation. Today, online databases allow for quick sorting of known reactions. Just like a player might remember and pass along certain formulae that they stumbled upon to solve elements of the Rubik's cube, so too chemists find trusted pathways and add their discoveries to the corporate knowledge base. In this way, the combined efforts of thousands of chemists can lead to significant innovations in chemical synthesis. Nevertheless, the process is almost always quite slow, and in some cases, the resulting hormone synthesis creates such low yields that it is cost prohibitive to manufacture them artificially.

Synthetic Analogues—Close Copies

Fortunately for the pharmaceutical industry, the universal presence of steroids in almost all life-forms means that they do not have to create the artificial synthesis in a laboratory to produce new steroids. The building blocks of many steroids may be collected or harvested relatively cheaply from certain plants and animals. While the human body relies on sophisticated organ systems to synthesize particular steroids, other organisms may achieve similar results through less specific means. For example, many corticosteroids are synthesized from metabolized progesterone. Commercially, pharmaceutical companies use similar molecules found in abundance in tomato plants (tomatidine) to replicate the characteristics of sapogenin steroids. These are fed to cows, which metabolize the tomatidine into progesterone, and this is then harvested through the animal waste (isolated from the urine and feces). Then, a variety of microorganisms are used to metabolize the progesterone into the desired corticosteroids. The use of steroid **analogues**, which are molecules that share similar structures to the original, and the use of **in vivo** metabolism (when you pass the material through another living organism) can at times result in a relatively inexpensive process—the animals and other organisms do most of the work.

Researchers try to uncover the synthesis pathways that transform one hormone molecule into another, in order to more easily identify commonly accessible analogues that will aid in more cost-effective industrial synthesis. This research is the backbone of the pharmaceutical industry. The use of synthetic analogues has both positive and negative implications. On the downside, the final product may only be an approximation of the original and not an exact copy, and as such, the actual chemical reaction may not exactly imitate the naturally derived metabolic process. On the upside, some of the artificial analogues may open new opportunities to further isolate desirable properties from the less desirable reactions. For example, most anabolic androgen steroids produce both tissue building (which strengthen certain muscle groups) and secondary sex characteristics (which define most female and male characteristics). A female bodybuilder may want stronger muscles, but may not want to sprout a beard. Some carefully synthesized analogues may strive to separate the anabolic functions (tissue growth) from the androgenic functions (sex hormones), to better manage the desired result. Understandably, this process is extremely difficult to guarantee and the results are not often predictable. These added risks, accompanied by new public demands, often create social and political pressures on the pharmaceutical industry that inevitably impacts the debates over appropriateness of steroid use both for therapeutic and performance enhancement objectives.

NONHORMONE STEROIDS

The four-ring gonane structure common to all steroids allows the possibility of thousands of different substituents and, therefore, thousands of different steroids, all of which makes classification difficult. Since the

Gonane (17 carbon atoms)

Estrane (18 carbon atoms) estrogens

Androstane (19 carbon atoms) androgens

Pregnane (21 carbon atoms) progesterone corticosteroids

Cholane (24 carbon atoms) bile acids

Cholestane (27 carbon atoms) cholestrol

(Courtesy of Brandon Fetterly)

1950s, biochemists began to classify steroids based on the number of carbon atoms on the commonly associated substituents on the gonane. Under this system, five main divisions emerged: cholestanes (with 27 carbons), cholic acids (with 24 carbons), pregnanes (with 21 carbons), androstanes (with 19 carbons), and estranes (with 18 carbons). Some of these were discovered in the later part of the 19th century, while others were only correctly identified during the mid-20th century. Within these broader classifications, hundreds—in some cases, thousands—of steroidal variations may be identified. As chemists develop more synthesis pathways, using a greater variety of analogue sources, the opportunity to create **synthetic hormones**, which are designer steroids based on theoretical modeling rather than natural occurrence, becomes much more common. In this way, the number of steroid options becomes even greater. For this section, we first discuss the nonhormonal steroids (cholestanes and cholic acids) and classify them according to their molecular composition. Second, we discuss the hormonal steroids (pregnanes, androstanes, and estranes), but in doing so it will be more useful to distinguish according to function (catabolic vs. anabolic) rather than molecular composition.

Cholestanes

The chemical structure of **cholestanes** begins with the core steroid gonane, and includes a substituent chain at the 17th carbon atom and two methyl groups very near to the gonane skeletal core. As the largest compound with 27 carbon atoms, cholestanes often act as a source from which other steroid types are derived. Some of the more significant derivatives of cholestanes include glycosides, saponins, benzoic acids, secosteroids (also known as vitamin D), and sterols. None of the cholestanes act directly as hormones, but most of them serve as precursors to hormones, and are therefore quite important to the pharmaceutical industry as key ingredients for both in vitro and in vivo synthesis.

Glycosides: Glycosides are found in a wide variety of plants and other organisms, and they serve an important function in pharmaceuticals. Glycosides affect hormone-producing tissues and produce yields that separate sugars and nonsugars. The cardiac glycosides are used extensively in medicines to treat heart disease because they effect the contraction of heart muscles. These steroids are most commonly harvested from foxglove, a purple flowering biennial shrub. The plant was identified as being useful to treat heart conditions as early as 1785 by Englishman William Withering. The group of drugs extracted from foxglove is named after its Latin title *Digitalus purpurea* and are collectively known as digitalin.

Saponins: Another type of glycosides extracted from plants are saponins, which are named for their characteristic foaming reaction when placed in water—the Latin word, *sapo*, means soap. The class of plants under the genus *saponaria* contains a saponin analogue that includes an additional nitrogen atom, and has historically been used as a main ingredient for making soap. These *saponaria*-based analogues are harmless to humans, but are toxic to cold-blooded animals due to the added nitrogen. This characteristic was recognized hundreds of years ago by certain indigenous populations and used as a fish poison—not to kill fish indiscriminately, but as a simpler way of harvesting fish. More importantly for the pharmaceutical industry, saponins also have anti-inflammatory properties. When introduced into the bloodstream, they can trigger hemolysis, which is the breakdown of red blood cells by separating hemoglobin from plasma resulting in the release of oxygen. Sapogenin compounds are extracted from pea or corn seeds, and then used as a starting material for the industrial manufacturing of numerous catabolic hormones, particularly the corticosteroids.

Benzoic acid: Benzoic acid was discovered in the mid-16th century and described most notably by the famous prognosticator Nostradamus, who extracted the compound from gum benzoin, which is a sap taken from certain trees in Asia. Of course, Nostradamus had no idea of its chemical structure and used it as a food preservative. Its molecular structure was discovered in the early 1830s by German scientists Justus von Liebig and Friedrich Wöhler. By the end of the 1800s, the antifungal properties of benzoic acid were identified and used to preserve fruits. More recently, chemists discovered pathways for in vitro synthesis cheaply and in mass quantities without the need of harvesting the sap from trees. American production amounts to 132,000 tons per year, and is used mostly by pharmaceutical companies and other industries. Benzoic acid is also a precursor to **anthranilic acid**, also known as vitamin L, which is itself a precursor to the tryptophan amino acid that is an essential part of the human diet. Tryptophan is a very common supplement among bodybuilders and often accompanies an anabolic steroid routine. Anthranilic acids, however, are also a precursor to the synthesis of the sedative methaqualone (commonly known as Quaalude), and as such are treated as a Class I chemical by the Federal Drug Enforcement Agency.

Secosteroids: Like many of the other cholestanes, secosteroids were discovered first as a practical compound long before it was recognized as a chemical steroid. **Vitamin D** was identified in the 1920s as an important cure for **rickets**, which is a disease that causes bone and cartilage tissues to fail in higher life-forms (human and animal). Softened bones respond to outside forces, such as gravity and heavy walking, often resulting in bent bones and even fractures. The disease is most frequently associated with malnutrition, and most often seen in children. It is due mostly to deficiency of calcium during bone growth. Vitamin D does not directly address the symptoms, but it does aid in the metabolism of calcium, which removes the fundamental cause of rickets. The discovery in 1921 by American researcher Elmer McCollum was followed almost immediately by Alfred Fabian Hess who showed that sunlight was most responsible for the synthesis of vitamin D. That same year, an American professor from the University of Wisconsin, Harry Steenbock, developed a process for passing milk under ultraviolet light resulting in vitamin D fortified milk. Steenbock patented the method, and within a generation rickets had largely disappeared among western cultures. The chemical structure of vitamin D was not discovered until later in the decade, when it was categorized as a sterol. Since then, vitamin D has been further divided into five different forms (D_1 to D_5), each distinguished by the molecular bonds in their side chains. Isolating pure forms of vitamin D is difficult, but pharmaceutical companies rely on in vivo synthesis to produce the starting materials, which are then further manipulated for more specific applications. Vitamin D is used in treatments for bone health, immunity disorders, influenza, cancer, and cardiovascular diseases.

Sterols: Perhaps, the most important subsets of cholestanes are the **sterols**, which are found in the tissues of virtually all life-forms—plant and animal (with the exception of some forms of algae and bacteria). On a molecular level, the common characteristic of sterols is that they all have a hydroxyl isotope on the third carbon in the gonane core structure. In higher life-forms, sterols are most predominant as **cholesterol**, though other forms can coexist. Cellular membranes are made of cholesterol and the endocrine system relies on protein-covered packets of cholesterol (called **lipoproteins**) to send messages from one system to the next, which trigger various feedback loops. The outward surfaces of lipoproteins are water soluble, so they can travel through the blood stream without dissolving, but the internal material is fat soluble, which means they dissolve as they enter the cell membrane. Low-density lipoprotein packets (**LDL**), often called bad cholesterol, tend to build up on internal walls of the blood vessels and can potentially create a buildup in the arteries leading to heart disease. High-density lipoproteins (**HDL**) are often referred to as good cholesterol because they can collect the LDL packets and clean out artery pathways. Most of the popular discussions on cholesterol refer to this transmission of information packets, because that is how cholesterol presents the most risk to heart health. In terms of biochemistry, though, cholesterol's far more important function is in the strengthening of plasma membranes and its nature as a mother for all steroids (hormonal and nonhormonal). Cholesterol is essential to all life-forms, plant and animal, and it serves as a critical component to the human endocrine system.

CHOLESTEROL—GOOD OR BAD?

Cholesterol was first discovered in the late 18th century by François Poulletier de la Salle who isolated the material from gallstones and bile. In 1928, German researchers Heinrich Wieland and Adolf Windaus discovered the molecular structure of cholesterol and earned a Nobel Prize for their efforts. Since then, 13 Nobel Prizes have been awarded for discoveries associated with cholesterol. Synthesis of cholesterol was achieved in the early 1950s by Robert Woodward who published a 40-step process that was not economically feasible for in vitro industrial production, but which was nevertheless significant in identifying the pathway for future researchers. Pharmaceutical companies seeking to better manage cholesterol levels try to interfere with the synthesis process as it occurs in the body. For example, statin drugs such as Lipitor, Mevacor, Zocor, Lescol, and Pravachol lower cholesterol levels by preventing the synthesis of mevalonate, which is a necessary acid used to synthesize cholesterol.

Virtually all steroid hormones, the vitamin D group, and cholic acids begin with cholesterol, which is broken down by various organ tissues to produce pregnanes, androstanes, and estranes. In terms of overall metabolism, cholesterol is significant because it serves as the source for both anabolic and catabolic hormones. Yet, therein lay the source of some controversy within the scientific community. On one hand, endocrinologists recognize cholesterol as an extremely important molecule necessary for the construction of plasma membranes and as the mother steroid from which all steroid hormones are formed—both in their final synthesis and their precursor protein forms. On the other, cardiologists point to the transmission of cholesterol packets (LDL, especially) as a significant cause of plaque buildup in the arteries, which is strongly associated with heart disease. Of course, these kinds of debates rarely limit themselves to the laboratory halls because federal research grants, public education campaigns, and federal nutrition guidelines all have a direct—often financial—impact on related pharmaceutical, academic, and agricultural industries.

Cholic Acids

Molecularly similar to cholestanes, the **cholane** (more commonly known as **cholic acids**) steroids share the same gonane structure but include a smaller substituent chain with three fewer carbon atoms (24 instead of 27). In the human body, cholic acids are synthesized from cholesterol by the liver and excreted as bile in the gall bladder and large intestines to help break down foods into their soluble fats so they can be reabsorbed in the lower intestines. These acids can be found in almost all vertebrates, and were isolated for practical purposes since ancient times. Chinese tradition held oxen bile as a natural anti-inflammatory, and modern research seems to confirm the potential that cholanes may influence the immune system to promote healing in localized inflammations. The chemical structure of cholic acids, however, was not discovered until the early 1940s. During the 1950s, researchers began to use deoxycholic acids (derived from oxen bile) as a detergent used to isolate certain soluble fat compounds. It is also synthesized for its **choleretic** properties, which stimulates the production and flow of bile in the liver, and for its **cholagogue** properties, which triggers the same process in the gall bladder. Both properties are used to treat digestive disorders and may also serve as a mild laxative.

HORMONE STEROIDS

When discussing nonhormone steroids, classification according to molecular composition is most convenient because it helps to emphasize the relative size of the steroid compounds and it shows the manner in which they can be synthesized into other smaller steroid forms. All the hormone steroids are relatively smaller in size (**pregnanes** with 21 carbons, **androstanes** with 19 carbons, and **estranes** with 18 carbons) than the cholestanes and as such they pass more easily through the cell membranes, which is an essential function of hormones in the endocrine system. Yet, more than their size and construction, it is the function of steroid hormones that is most significant in understanding their differences. Some steroids help to build up cell tissues (anabolic) and others help to break down or convert cell tissues (catabolic).

The molecular size of steroids is important because it impacts the speed by which they pass through the associated cell membranes, but the chemical names for these categories can be confused with the functional operations when we come to the pregnane class. Pregnane steroids are made up of 21 carbons and like cholesterol from which it is derived they can serve as a source material for four distinct types of steroids, both anabolic and catabolic. The starting pregnane molecule derived after cholesterol is broken down in the adrenal cortex is **pregnenolone**, and this serves as a parent molecule for all hormone steroids, including progestogins, androgens, and estranes. **Progestogins** are sex-related hormones and anabolic in nature. Yet that same 21-carbon skeletal structure is also the basis for a group of catabolic steroid hormones that include mineralocorticoids and glucocorticoids.

Even though the synthesis pathway for corticosteroids may begin with a progestogin, the two hormone groups are functionally quite different. For the purposes of functional classification, progestogins (an anabolic steroid that builds up tissues) should not be confused with mineralocorticoids or glucocorticoids (catabolic steroids that break down tissues). To avoid this confusion, we refer to the catabolic half of steroids in the pregnane molecular group as **corticosteroids**. Corticosteroids are responsible for regulating metabolism, immunity, and also influencing memory functions. The anabolic half of the pregnane molecular group (the progestogins) as well as the andrane and estrange molecular groups are collectively referred to as **sex steroids**. They are mainly responsible for the building of cellular tissues, reproduction, and the secondary sex characteristics.

Corticosteroids

The corticoid steroids are so named for their association with the adrenal cortex. This connection was first discovered in the mid-19th century by Thomas Addison, who noticed a correlation between diseased adrenal glands and symptoms related to salt cravings, low blood sugar, weakness, weight loss, and low blood pressure. The adrenal glands produce both kinds of catabolic hormones that regulate salt and sugar content in our body. The salt (mostly sodium), electrolyte, and water balances in the body are regulated by a group of steroids known as **mineralocorticoids** (mineral refers to the regulation of inorganic materials such as sodium and potassium, and corticoid refers to their association with the adrenal cortex). The sugar (mostly glucose) balances are regulated by **glucocorticoid** steroids. Together, they are called corticosteroids, and they play a significant role in metabolism and immunity, and researchers are beginning to discover connections in the cerebral cortex that influence memory function.

Mineralocorticoids: In the human body, the primary mineralocorticoid steroid hormone is **aldosterone**, which is synthesized in the adrenal cortex and sent to the kidneys, where it is largely responsible for regulating electrolyte levels, blood pressure, and volume. This steroid was isolated in the early 1950s by American researchers James Tait and Sylvia Simpson. It is part of a complex feedback system called the **renin-angiotensin-aldosterone cascade** that begins with the release of enzymes triggered by low sodium levels in the blood. These enzymes activate other latent peptide hormones resident in the kidneys (angiotensin I/II), which in turn increase the level of potassium in the blood stream and also triggers the release of aldosterone from the adrenal cortex. Aldosterone uses the bloodstream to reach the kidneys, where it aids in the absorption of the sodium and the secretion of potassium and hydrogen ions into the urine. The added sodium attracts water molecules and increases the blood pressure and volume.

As a catabolic steroid, the nature of aldosterone is to break down and absorb; too much aldosterone can lead to excessive sodium absorption, leading to water retention and higher blood pressure (**hypertension**). It could also increase excretion of potassium, which may lead to muscle loss and paralysis. At the same time, too little aldosterone can lead to similar effects. **Addison's Disease** is characterized by muscle weakness, drowsiness, weight loss, and other skin and gastrointestinal disturbances. Other symptoms include headaches, muscle spasms and numbness, constipation or frequent urination, and excessive thirst. Pharmaceutical companies use aldosterone, or its analogues, to manage swelling (edema) and to treat immune system disorders.

Glucocorticoids: The glucocorticoid steroids were first isolated and synthesized on a commercial scale in the late 1940s, and include four permutations of 11-deoxycortisol, cortisterone, cortisone, and cortisol. This steroid hormone group is produced by the adrenal cortex, but it impacts almost every system in the body because they play a critical role in the conversion of glucose, fat, and proteins into energy used by almost all cell types. They also play a role in activating the immune system. As such, glucocorticoid steroids have an impact on energy levels, inflammation, and allergic reactions.

As a metabolic agent, **cortisol** enhances the expression of enzymes to facilitate **gluconeogenesis** in the liver. The liver is a very large organ that acts as a filter for the blood, which passes from multiple points in the digestive tract through thousands of large and small capillaries before being sent through to the heart and brain. In the process, the liver both stores and releases energy by breaking down proteins, fats, and sugars through the synthesis and activation of virtually all steroid forms (cholestanes, cholic acids, corticosteroids, and precursors for appropriate sex steroids). Gluconeogenesis occurs when glucose is synthesized, and **glycolysis** is the process during which glucose is broken down into its intermediate parts—thus storing and releasing energy. The brain is especially dependent on glucose, since it cannot use fats or proteins for energy. Too little cortisol can starve the brain, resulting in hypoglycemic symptoms such as tremors, anxiety, weakness, blurred vision, and even coma and seizures. Cortisol plays a role in memory functions, and has an impact on learning and mood. Other research suggests cortisol deficiencies may be associated with a variety of psychological disorders that seem to imitate symptoms of post-traumatic stress disorder and may contribute to chemical addictions in an attempt to address the deficiency. By contrast, too much cortisol can lead to hyperglycemia and **Cushing's Syndrome**, which is characterized by fat deposits in the neck, trunk, and face; thinning of the skin leading to bruises and purplish striae in the abdomen; high blood pressure; and other emotional effects, such as depression, insomnia, and loss of libido.

Balancing Risks and Benefits of Cortisol Therapies

Glucocorticoid steroids also play a significant role in the immune system. In the mid-1940s, Dr. Philip Hench noticed that his patients with rheumatoid arthritis often found relief during pregnancy, which is when the body significantly increases its cortisol production. Hench began proscribing cortisol to his rheumatoid arthritis patients and noticed significant relief of their symptoms. He and two other doctors shared a Nobel Prize for this discovery in 1950, and their success triggered a revival in steroid research. In 1955, two pharmaceutical companies (Schering Corporation and the Upjohn Company) released a synthetic form of cortisol called **prednisone**, which were sold in tablet form under the brand names of Meticorten and Delta-Cortef. They were used as an anti-inflammatory, but by the end of the decade, researchers began to see unintended side effects from long-term use.

Inflammation is a natural byproduct of our body's immune system. When a foreign substance (such as bacteria or a virus) is detected in the bloodstream, white blood cells (known as **leukocytes**) are produced from the white bone marrow as a natural defense mechanism. These leukocytes are drawn to the problem to fight (literally cover and destroy) the foreign cells, and this action can result in redness and warmth in the effected spot as well as swelling and pain. Cortisol works by turning off the enzymes, receptors, and genes that are responsible for releasing the white blood cells. Prednisone was developed in tablet form, which means it always resulted in **systemic** reactions because the steroid enters the blood stream and affects the entire body. Systemic use of glucocorticoid steroids will inhibit immune systems everywhere, including those that are not inflamed and those that serve necessary protections against other diseases. System immune suppression leaves patients susceptible to a variety of ailments. In addition, cortisol still has an impact on metabolism even when it is intended only to address immune issues. Excessive amounts of cortisol can produce harsh side effects on the body's metabolism, resulting in high blood pressure and psychological mood swings. It is also linked to diabetes.

During the 1960s, pharmaceutical companies sought out an analogue synthesis to cortisol that would increase the inflammatory properties while reducing these unwanted side effects. Many synthetic steroids were produced, but the most significant innovation in this area came from a more localized application of the corticosteroids. Researchers developed a spray form of the steroid in the early 1970s, which allowed asthma patients to inhale the cortisol analogue, passing it directly to the lungs. Most asthma related disorders result from inflammation of the bronchial tubes that restrict airways, and direct application of the steroid reduced inflammation locally without affecting other immune systems. Asthma is a significant health problem that affects the lives and well-being of people all over the world, and the introduction of the asthma inhaler led to rapid expansion in corticosteroid applications, including other forms of localized applications such as topical solutions and localized injections.

Today, steroid inhalers can be divided between those that offer quick relief lasting only 3 or 4 hours, or those offering extended relief for 12 hours. Short-term steroid inhalers include formoterol (sold as Foradil and Oxis) and salmeterol (sold as Serevent). Extended term steroid inhalers include beclometasone (sold as Beclazone and Qvar), budesonide (sold as

Pulmicort), fluticasone (sold as Flovent), mometasone (sold as Asmanex), and ciclesonide (sold as Alvesco). Corticosteroids are among the most proscribed drugs in the world. Doctors prescribe synthetic corticosteroids to treat a broad spectrum of immunity disorders, including inflammation, asthma, allergies, shock, neoplastic disorders (tumor growth), and collagen diseases (like rheumatoid arthritis). Metabolic disorders, including adrenocortical deficiencies, are still being treated with cortisol, but the greatest amount of research focuses on its anti-inflammatory properties.

Corticosteroids are clearly designed to serve therapeutic purposes. There is, nevertheless, some room for controversy in their use. With few exceptions, corticosteroids mostly treat the symptoms of inflammation, but they do not necessarily address the cause of the disorders. Despite the significant research into synthetic analogues that enhance the preferred properties and strive to diminish the negative side effects, there remains no perfect solution. Physicians debate the medical ethics of whether the benefits of short-term relief outweigh the possible risks of long-term usage. Moreover, there are sociopolitical issues related to the intertwining roles of the pharmaceutical industry, government and public policy, and individual demand in promoting a drug culture that encourages expectations of short-term gratification at the expense of long-term solutions.

Sex Steroids

The sex steroid hormones are so named because they are responsible for facilitating the operation of the sex organs (gonads) and for the development of those physical characteristics that most distinguish men and women (known as **secondary sex traits**). Some of these characteristics include deeper voice and presence of facial hair on men, relatively smoother skin on women, the enlargement of certain sex organs on both genders, and the relative differences in size, strength, and physical endurance. Aside from unchangeable differences in bone structure and the chromosome chain (XX vs. XY), most of the physiological distinctions between men and women are determined by the predominant presence of male steroid hormones (mostly testosterone) and female steroid hormones (mostly progesterone and estradiol). Each of these sex steroid groups are molecularly varied, ranging from 18 to 21 carbon atoms, which is important in terms of biochemical synthesis. The larger progestin steroids (with 21 carbons) are broken down to form the androgen steroids (with 19 carbons), which in turn are broken down further to form the estrane steroids (with 18 carbons). It also means, though, that a little of each sex steroid must be present to some degree in both males and females. It is the ratio and dominance of one kind over another than sustains the outward sex differences between genders.

As would be expected, the overall **steroidogenesis** process for sex steroids is unique for each gender, but the first step begins in the same place for men and women, the adrenal cortex. The adrenal cortex is a tiny organ but it is divided into three parts, where each of the three hormone types is synthesized from the common parent molecule, pregnenolone. One section (called the *zona glomerulosa*) synthesizes the mineralocorticoids like aldosterone to be sent as needed out to the kidneys and elsewhere. Another section (called the *zona fasciculata*) synthesizes the glucocorticoids like cortisol that is sent to the liver and brain. The last section (called the *zona reticularis*) is responsible for synthesizing the androgens, which are sent to the respective gonads of each gender. For all these sections, the adrenal cortex first takes cholesterol and turns it into pregnenolone. It is from the pregnenolone structure that other steroids are created. This process is not reversible, but there is a feedback loop within the adrenal cortex that helps to limit the rate of production.

The adrenal cortex usually ends its synthesis of sex steroids after pregnenolone is converted into **androstenedione**, which is then converted easily into both testosterone and estrone. Both molecules are found in men and women and are used for various parts of the body that are not directly related to reproduction. Testosterone is converted to **dihydrotestosterene** (DHT), which is used for building muscle tissue. Estrone is converted into estradiol, which is used for building adipose tissues (fat tissues). Since estradiol is synthesized from testosterone, the sex steroids for both men and women are often referred to generically as **androgens**. In Greek, the word *andros* means man and *gennao* means to produce; so androgen refers to the production of man. On a molecular level, though, the male steroids have 19 carbon atoms and are called androstanes, and their steroids (testosterone and its precursors) are called androgens. Female steroids have only 18 carbon atoms, and its steroids (estrone and estradiol) are called **estrogens**.

Biochemical Differences between Men and Women

Sexual differentiation begins mostly in the gonads. In women, the ovaries synthesize their own **estrone** steroid, which are the 18-carbon molecules mostly associated with the sexual reproduction and secondary sex characteristics of women. The ovaries contain unique cells (called *theca* and *granulosa*), which can synthesize cholesterol directly into pregnenolone and then into estrone and **estradiol**, which is secreted through follicles in the ovaries. After ovulation, the same cells produce progesterone, which is used to prepare the uterus for implantation of the ovum. The synthesis of estradiol may also occur outside the ovaries.

In men, the testes are mostly responsible for synthesizing **testosterone**, but like the ovaries, they also synthesize small amounts of other steroids. Within the testes, **Leydig cells** convert cholesterol into pregnenolone, then to androstenedione, and then to testosterone, which is also converted into DHT and estradiol. For both men and women, these steroids may be synthesized locally elsewhere, but the testes ensure that the vast majority of androgen steroids are in the form of testosterone, while the ovaries ensure that most of its steroids end up as estradiol.

Anabolic Steroids as Contraceptives

Beginning in the 1950s, researchers began searching for progesterone analogues in an attempt to regulate the ovulation cycle, which in turn would result in a chemical-based artificial contraceptive. By 1957, Gregory Pincus, John Rock, and Christopher Tietze combined existing synthetic analogues of progesterone and estradiol into a single pill, which they described as an **anovulent**, which means that it prevents ovulation and thereby prevents conception. The drug was originally approved by the Food and Drug Administration (FDA) as a tool for addressing menstrual disorders and infertility, but it was given additional approval in 1960 as the world's first oral contraceptive. A little more than a decade later, the FDA approved a synthetic progesterone analogue that increased the thickness of the uterus so much that it served as a barrier to the ovum, thereby achieving the same contraceptive result. Since then, dozens of other synthetic analogues have been developed for the purposes of contraception, or to serve as postcoital abortifaciants. Their delivery mechanisms now range from tablet form, injections, patches, and subcutaneous implants, which are marketed by dozens of different pharmaceutical companies.

There has been significant controversy associated with the development of these synthetic steroid hormones for the purposes of artificial contraception. The most critical reason stems from the fact that these steroid hormones, unlike the corticosteroids analogues, deal with the creation of new human life. From a moral perspective, there are serious questions about the right of individuals to prevent or destroy life that might begin at the first moment of conception. On the other side of the argument are those who see artificial contraception as a critical part of female liberation and gender equity. Removing the fear of unintended pregnancies may extend greater opportunities for women in the workplace. The determination of when life begins, how precious it should be treated, and the guidelines for the protection of its prenatal development do not lie with scientific reasoning alone. At heart, these are religious and philosophical questions and the answers reflect deeply held beliefs on both sides of the issue. Aside from the obvious questions of defining the moment of life, there are other ethical questions about the wisdom of separating the consequences (conception and birth) from the actions which carries with it a great deal of other added emotional and psychological ramifications (sexual relationships). In addition, there are a great number of sociopolitical issues related to the role of government, public financing, consumer protection, public education, and industrial responsibility that are all intertwined with the invention and hormone-based contraceptives. Perhaps more than any other steroid-related issue, the synthetic manipulation of estrogen and progesterone inspired cultural debates that transformed the course of political and social history.[1]

Anabolic Steroids as Ergogenic

Of course, the development of synthetic analogues for male androgen steroids has experienced only marginally less controversy. Since the most noticeable secondary sex characteristics in males are the increases in muscle strength and endurance, synthetic forms of testosterone were pursued for their performance-enhancing properties shortly after discovery. Testosterone was first isolated and synthesized in the mid-1930s by German chemists Adolf Butenandt and Leopold Ruzicka, who both shared a Nobel Prize for the discovery in 1937. Because the scientists were German, later observers theorized that the first use of synthetic testosterone for performance-enhancing purposes occurred during World War II when Hitler gave the drugs to his Nazi soldiers. There is little evidence to support this claim, but it is a very popular speculation because the central attraction of synthetic testosterone is that it will increase strength and lead to a scientifically designed *überman*, which seems to fit right in line with the themes of Nazi propaganda. The fundamental controversy behind the synthetic production of male sex steroids lay mostly in their unintended health risks, which give rise to concerns of competitive fairness and maintaining integrity within each sport.

---

1. For a more in-depth discussion of birth control and its related issues, please see Aharon W. Zorea, *Birth Control*, New York: ABC-CLIO/Greenwood Press, 2012.

The more documented historical anecdotes of early testosterone synthesis suggest that the prospect of performance enhancement followed closely on the heels of research originally intended for therapeutic purposes. There are more than a few testimonials indicating that state sponsored Olympic Teams began to experiment with various anabolic analogues as early as the late 1940s. By the mid-1950s, John Ziegler, an American research chemist who also served as a consultant for the U.S. Olympic Weight Lifting Team, developed **methandrostenalone**, which was a synthetic version of androstenedione. His research lab, Ciba Pharmaceuticals, marketed the drug as a treatment for hypogonadism in 1958 under the name of Dianabol. Yet, from the start, its use was primarily directed to athletes. Ziegler is credited with creating the first legal androgen-based steroid, but anecdotal evidence suggests that the unregulated use of such drugs may have been popular among select professional athletes around the world throughout the 1950s. The International Olympic Committee did not formally prohibit the use of steroids as performing enhancers until 1975.

WHAT IS THE DIFFERENCE BETWEEN ERGOGENIC DRUGS, PEDS, AND STEROIDS?

The term ergogenic means performance enhancing. The acronym PED is short for performance-enhancing drugs. Ergogenic drugs (or PEDs) may include any number of drugs beyond anabolic steroids, so either option is usually preferred over the generic term steroids. Since modern society may not always understand ergogenic, most sports writers use the term PED in the news stories.

The Industry of Ergogenic Drugs

The number of legally and illegally available forms of **ergogenic** steroids developed since the 1950s is not easily known, but there are at least 600 anabolic androgens and likely hundreds more of various analogues synthesized for every androgen-based steroid precursor. The commercial and competitive natures of the sports industry fuel a constant demand for chemical supplements that enhance the secondary male sex characteristics of strength, endurance, and rapid healing. The public and private sectors have reacted to these demands accordingly. Since the 1970s and 1980s, governing agencies of almost all professional and amateur sports associations have initiated safeguards against the use of anabolic andro-genic steroids and other performance enhancers in an attempt to protect the integrity of their competitive records and achievements. Nevertheless, sports scandals revealing illegal steroid use have emerged frequently in al-most every sport since the 1990s.

Policymakers and legislatures in local and federal governments have enacted guidelines and prohibitions against certain drugs to protect the public health, but new analogues are routinely being created and these drugs are not always recognized as ergogenic until they become associated with a particular scandal. More importantly, even though the public reacts harshly to each new revelation of scandal, there is nonetheless strong pres-sure among consumers for more interesting and competitive sports play. This creates mutually reinforcing tensions between public demand for in-creasingly competitive sports forums, the pharmaceutical industry's desire to meet that demand, and the government's desire to regulate production and safeguard public health. In the scientific community, there is a sort of race between competing industries: on the one side are researchers trying to develop more effective ways of detecting the presence of performance-enhancing drugs, while on the other side there are researchers trying to de-velop more effective drugs that escape detection.

The Morality of Aging

In addition to the issues related to fair competition and public safety, there are other distinguishing characteristics of sex steroids that lead to larger moral and philosophical dilemmas. Among the steroid hormone classes, only the sex steroids appear to be specifically age dependent. The corticosteroids and nonhormone steroids are produced according the indi-vidual feedback mechanisms within each person's physiological profile. After maturity, the internal synthesis of steroids does not greatly vary ac-cording to how old you are. For example, decreases in the amounts of cho-lic acid, or aldosterone, or cortisol are due to degenerative failure of the respective organs, but not due to any natural or anticipated life-cycle arc. By contrast, the sex hormones follow a very definite age-related pattern. Production begins at very low levels shortly after birth and gradually in-creases during the first third of a typical life span, before tabling off during the next third, and finally gradually diminishing back to low levels again toward the end of life. In essence, the ability to bear and raise children fol-lows a predefined window with the natural life cycle.

What is not clear, though, is whether the natural aging process causes this life cycle or whether the life cycle is responsible for the outward signs of aging. There are certainly strong indications that other systems in the body experience natural catabolic changes over the life cycle, with the general observation that systems become frailer and more likely to fail as they age. But it is not clear whether those changes are due to predefined schedules or if they reflect the systemic reductions in the anabolic activators that would otherwise keep them vibrant. We certainly get old, but do we have to? There is some scientific debate over this, which leads to a number of philosophical issues related to the scientific possibility of a "fountain of youth." Each side of the question carries with it implications on the relative efficacy of long-term strategies for maintaining wellness. In addition, there are other sociopolitical issues related to the appropriateness of extending activities of youth into old age. It also leads to eugenic-like questions related to whether or not science is able to, or should even try to, create a more perfect human through careful hormonal manipulation.

CONCLUSION

Who is the final authority in deciding whether the drug is safe or harmful to individuals? If an anabolic steroid is used as a general supplement to fight aging, but is not necessarily used to treat a specific ailment, then is it a therapeutic tool or a cosmetic tool? Should individuals be allowed to voluntarily accept the risky side effects of a steroid as long as they also provide the desired effects of increased performance or youthful vigor? What are the ethical differences between a carefully prescribed diet, a synthetic dietary supplement, a pre-steroidal supplement, and a customized anabolic steroid? Who is to determine the lines that distinguish each and the degree to which they impact competitive fairness? Is this a matter for individuals to decide, for the government to mandate, or for sports associations to regulate? These and other questions emerge whenever any drug is developed for their ability to enhance, rather than for their therapeutic potential to treat specific physiological disorders.

In the next two chapters, we examine with more detail the social and political history of how the public has both encouraged and reacted against developments in steroid research. Chapter Two first considers the role of research into catabolic steroids and their potential therapeutic use. Special emphasis will be given to the role of steroid research in the development of a chemical culture in contemporary American society. Chapter Three then discusses the history of popular demand and public reaction to anabolic steroid research intended for performance enhancement. Special emphasis will be directed to the role of steroid use in the increasing expectations of physical perfection.

CHAPTER 2

Historical Background of Therapeutic Steroids

In 1990, Carl Djerassi published his first of several autobiographies under the title *Steroids Made it Possible*. Djerassi was a biochemist who was involved in the very early synthesis of steroids in the late 1940s and early 1950s. His work on the progestin **norethindrone** at the start of the decade was the first analogue synthesis of progesterone that could be taken orally and still remain effective. Though Djerassi's team initially intended the drug as a form of pest control to prevent animals from breeding, it was later embraced by a working group financed by Planned Parenthood and led by John Rock as the basis for the first oral contraceptive for women. Djerassi's pharmaceutical company, Syntex Laboratories, later marketed the drug after the Food and Drug Administration (FDA) approval in 1960.

Djerassi intended the title of his autobiography as a sort of tongue-in-cheek admission of what he most owed his wealth and fortune to. In his later years, after a series of inventions and awards in numerous fields, Djerassi converted his large northern California cattle ranch into an artist colony and named it SMIP—Steroids Made it Possible. The acronym could just as easily be read as Syntex Made it Possible, but his autobiography chose to identify his field of research and not his corporate holdings. Djerassi freely admitted that he never intended to develop a human contraceptive when he first synthesized norethindrone. He reflected, "Not in our wildest dreams . . . did we imagine" the synthetic progestin drug would be used on humans. Nevertheless, his patent on the drug earned him the title "Father of the Pill," which also earned him a great deal of money. Djerassi attributed his later successes, in large part, to his initial research into steroids. Throughout his very long career, which included more than 1,200 scientific publications and numerous inventions, steroid research always held a central place.

At the same time, though, Djerassi's autobiographical reflection might also be a suitable description of another larger historical shift in biochemical research that came to dominate the 20th century. Research into steroid synthesis was not the only avenue for scientific exploration after the Second World War, but it certainly lead the way in stimulating the search for chemical solutions to medical ailments. During the early part of the century, the pharmaceutical industry mainly played a small role in the larger story of industrialization. Chemical manufacturers focused much of their research on application for factory use, cosmetics, and agricultural production. After the war, drug companies shifted their attention toward new synthetic chemical compounds for treating the underlying causes of medical disorders rather than just the symptoms. Pharmacology earned a place of equal if not greater importance than surgery, and the pharmaceutical industry became a dominant force in defining the direction of health care.

The success of the therapeutic use of chemistry became obvious by the 1960s, resulting in a cultural reaction that both welcomed and warned about the growing chemical culture. On the one hand, the scientific community played a major role in providing new hope for those who suffered ailments that seemed to have no solution. On the other hand, there were obvious concerns as drugs were used and abused for recreational purposes, and the balance between short-term benefit and long-term costs became blurred. Among the young, especially, this balance was challenged, and as that generation now reaches its seniority, the impact on American culture is strongly felt.

OF MAGIC, HOLISTIC REMEDY, AND OTHER PRESCIENTIFIC APPROACHES TO MEDICINE

The use of chemical medicines begins nearly 4,000 years ago in ancient Egypt, when medical treatments occurred at localized temples and health care was the responsibility of priests. From a modern perspective, their list of remedies might seem quaint, but the exhaustive lists used to treat ailments reflect a systematic approach to health care that was not accidental or random. Ancient Egyptian documents testify to a wide variety of treatment options, including oral consumption, topical salves, and suppositories (which act as a temporary internal application). Much of the West's understanding of herb lore came from such systematic tables of ailments and their associated herbal treatments developed by Egyptian doctors: thyme provided pain relief; mixtures of dill, balsam, apples, onions,

and parsley served as a laxative; bad breath was cured by mint and cara-
way seeds; headaches resolved with aloe and poppy seeds; burns or other
skin rashes treated with aloe; and dozens of other concoctions were linked
to specific cures.

BIOCHEMISTRY IN ANCIENT EGYPT?

Though most of Egypt's medical treatment came in the form of magical incantations, there is some indication that the Egyptians stumbled upon more
than a few chemical interactions, if only by accident. For example, modern doctors would still recommend aloe vera as a treatment for burns and
other skin disorders because its gel contains polysaccharides and a host of
amino acids and sterols (particularly lupol, campesterol, and β-sitosterol).
Topical application to effected cells stimulates macrophases and fibroblasts
that increase collagen and proteoglycan synthesis leading to tissue repair.
Not surprisingly, the Egyptian records do not make any references to these
interactions. Similarly, the poppy seeds remedy for headache is reasonable
because it contains pantothenic acid, linoleic acid, and diacetylmorphine.
The codeine and morphine content triggers the release of endorphins (endogenous opioid peptides) from the pituitary gland throughout the central
nervous system to produce an euphoric, analgesic effect. Again, there was
no mention of these chemical reactions in the Egyptian lists. Instead, the ancient writings always included incantations that the priest and patient would
recite together according to special formulae, and thereby elicit the aid of
specific gods and goddess that were ultimately responsible for the cure. The
ancient treatments may not be unusual to us now, but the ancient understanding of their efficacy certainly is.

In practice, it is quite likely that the Egyptians discovered these remedies after many years of anecdotal observations that connected the in-
gestion of specific herbs with certain associated responses. But, in their
ignorance of the molecular operations of human physiology, they attributed these correlations to divine interventions. Indeed, the Egyptians believed that there were special gods responsible for the healthy operation
of every observable part of the body and still more deities who served as
overseers to those gods. The herbs were not special in themselves, except
when used in conjunction with the appropriate spell. They were seen as
magical reagents that were activated by secret incantations known by a
selected order of religious priests. In ancient times, then, health care was
divined by a mix of observation, tradition, and superstition.

Humanist Medicine: Passive Observation

Around 2,500 years ago, the birth of humanism helped define the rising Greek civilization as natural philosophers severed the tie between superstition and science. Hippocrates earned the title "Father of Western Medicine" from his insistence that sickness and disease were due to natural, discernible causes and not due to the anger or whims of gods in the spiritual realm. Known for his unwearied observation of his patients, Hippocrates endeavored to consolidate all the available natural remedies together, remove the associated incantations, and then offered detailed descriptions of his observations as to their anticipated effect.

Though Hippocrates rejected divine intervention as a cause for typical ailments, he still held a pseudomystical view of the human body. Diseases, he argued, were the result of an unhealthy ratio of various liquids called humors that ruled over the functioning of human physiology. These liquids were controlled by the inhalation of vapors and were responsible

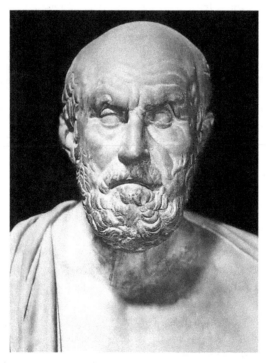

Hippocrates was a Greek physician born in 460 BC on the island of Cos, Greece. He became known as the founder of Western medicine and was regarded as the greatest physician of his time. (Library of Congress)

for health, mood, personality, and, to some extent, fate. Hippocrates and his later adherents maintained a supernatural explanation for the workings of human physiology. He broke the bond between medicine and superstition, but the very strong tradition of the almost magical operation of the human body persisted, leading doctors to observe more and accommodate rather than interfere and manipulate with the basic functioning of the human system.

NINETEENTH-CENTURY VIEW OF THE BODY

Legacies of Hippocrates's passive approach to health care can be seen even in the scientific age. As late as the mid-1800s, long after the invention of microscopes, dozens of so-called sex manuals were published by reputable doctors describing the anatomy of the human reproductive system. Dr. James Ashton's 1859 monograph, *The Book of Nature*, included detailed illustrations of the gonad system, with references to sperm, ovum, and very tiny ducts that are just beyond visibility with the human eye, all of which indicate an acute understanding of the physical operation of both male and female anatomy. Yet, Ashton's accompanying explanation of the reproductive process revealed presumptions that hearkened back to a premodern era. He clearly understood that joining sperm and ovum led to conception and he provided several alternate approaches for interfering with that process to ensure contraception. At the same time, he also described sperm as the source of male vitality, energy, intelligence, and strength. He wrote tales of Persian Princes with large harems containing hundreds of wives, who, due to their constant sexual activity, were weak, feeble minded, with low energy and poor decision-making abilities. Their sons were born likewise weak because the life force had been spent in too much activity. Excessive release or buildup of such vitality led to discernible psychological and emotional symptoms. Ashton was not unique in these beliefs and his recommendations were echoed by dozens of others well into the 1870s. It was not until just before the 20th century that this kind of commentary began to fade away in favor of more precise chemical explanations.

Modern Alternative Medicines

Even in the 21st century, it is possible to see traces and legacies of Hippocrates's mystical view of human physiology. The increasingly noticeable following of **alternative medical** approaches, in part, relies on the presumption that not all the operations of human physiology are (and can fully be) understood through the objective research methods of modern science. Often pointing to non-Western sources of authority, some of these approaches include homeopathy, naturopathy, energy therapies, and other regional traditions such as the Indian system of balancing humors called Ayurvedic medicine and the Chinese traditional system that manipulate life energy called Qi (or Chi). Each of these approaches contend that there are invisible forces—not just unseen as in ultamicroscopic, but also invisible as in not physically measurable—that control physical health, mental performance, and psychological and even spiritual well-being.

The efficacy of alternative medicine is difficult to measure by the quantitative standards of biochemical science. In part, this may be due to the **placebo effect**, which is the phenomenon that occurs when people believe that the treatment they are taking will produce the desired results. It is not magic, but the power of suggestion and the mind's willingness to experience positive changes has been demonstrably measured with predictable frequency. Though not thoroughly understood, the effect is so pervasive that researchers in both the hard and soft sciences must account for its presence whenever they design an experiment.

It is reasonable to expect that some people may find relief through nontraditional medicine simply because they believe it will do them some good. Unfortunately, the placebo effect also carries the risk of masking undesirable side effects that are chemically unavoidable, and which may cause internal harm that is not always obvious until the symptoms are so great that a solution is no longer available. Conversely, the placebo effect may also change direction without any logical reason. A baseball player, for example, may find genuine support from a lucky charm leading to a new winning streak. In the same way, though, the player may later believe that luck ran out, leading to a new slump. In either case, potential placebo effectiveness is not a dependable criterion for evaluating the relative value of a particular treatment option.

The approaches of alternate medicine necessarily rely on different measures for determining efficacy of any treatment, including various steroid-based supplements. At the same time, alternative medicine must coexist in modern society, which otherwise maintains a strong confidence in the traditional science—and often both approaches share common support. This incongruence may play a role in marketing health care remedies through mainstream media outlets. Traditional medicine encourages greater confidence in the ability to find a solution for an ailment—whether it is serious or trivial. Nontraditional medicine encourages hope for new and previously unrealized solutions that have not been fully recognized by traditional authorities. Together, both pressures coincide to provide legitimacy for a marketing campaign aiming to sell a dietary supplement.

Some of the steroid-based supplements intended for therapeutic use (not for bodybuilding) are marketed as an alternative medical solution. With such teasing taglines, such as "what your doctor does not want you know . . .," these marketing strategies rely on appeals to authorities that lay outside the traditional scientific community. Whether steroid based or not, nontraditional remedies provide a persistent countervailing pressure for decision making made by individuals, competitive associations, and public governance. At heart, these alternative traditions create some contrast (at times antagonistic and at times just dynamic tension) which helps to fuel the support for nonscientific basis of authority.

Of Science, Technology, and Social Engineering

The path of traditional medicine changed significantly as it passed through the scientific revolution of the 16th century, which when combined with a number of other sociopolitical changes ushered in the modern era. The humanistic renaissance within a monotheistic society encouraged more active search for material solutions for material causes. One God, one material order, and one law of nature awaited discovery through careful and systematic human observation and experimentation. Francis Bacon, following a long line of predecessors, presented a formal system for identifying, evaluating, and testing new knowledge, which is now referred to simply as the **scientific method**. The first critical component of Bacon's process was to gather a history of the subject and compile as many factual observations that existed into one list. From there, researchers would identify incongruities and formulate hypothesis for explaining them, which would then be tested and evaluated again until a more thorough understanding of the subject emerged.

Systematic Symptom Observations

Most of the medical advances made in the years prior to the 20th century emerged through a systematic categorization of symptoms and the observable treatment effects. This approach was more active than Hippocrates's passive accommodation approach, but they still focused on the identification of effects (symptoms) rather than on the more precise diagnosis of specific underlying causes. Louis Pasteur's innovations of the mid-1800s were extremely significant, but they were limited to recognizing correlations rather than detailed understanding of primary causes. His pasteurization process raised the temperature of liquids to a point that was sure to kill any hidden microorganisms, but it did not explain how those organisms actually attached themselves to the liquid molecules or how they transferred from host to host. This was true also of Pasteur's other important discovery of immunization.

While studying cholera in chickens, Pasteur isolated the bacteria and used it on live animals to test reactions. At one point, a batch of his cholera culture somehow failed and the infected chickens did not develop the disease. Pasteur later discovered that the chickens were no longer able to be infected, even when using more effective batches of cholera culture. Later experiments led Pasteur to conclude that the animals had developed some kind of immunity and this led him to create a vaccine for the anthrax disease in cattle. Pasteur's discovery served as a template for researchers around the world who used mild versions of an infectious disease to create vaccinations that strengthened the host's immune system to protect against further infection. Yet, critical as these discoveries were, they did not proceed from a specific understanding of how the diseases actually interacted within the immune system or how the vaccinations worked in creating a stronger immunity. The discoveries instead relied on systematic observations of a successful process.

Systematic Molecular Observations

What was lacking in Pasteur's research was a more thorough understanding of spatial relationship of molecular structures, how they interacted with organic and nonorganic materials, and the pathways of protein synthesis involved in human metabolism. These critical elements of molecular biology were not long in coming, and very shortly after Pasteur's time, they developed simultaneously during the industrial revolution of the late 19th and early 20th centuries. Jacob van't Hoff helped launch the field of **stereochemistry** by designing three-dimensional models of simple molecules in the 1870s, and in the 1890s Edward Buchner helped to launch the field of biochemistry with his discovery that inorganic yeast could extract sugar during fermentation even outside the living cells. Meanwhile, 20th-century innovations in metallurgy, electricity, and optics led to critical developments in X-ray diffraction and electron microscopy, which provided researchers with the tools for better isolating particular molecules. By the 1950s, these and other fields converged together, to reveal new depths of biological understanding that dipped below the larger expressions of classical biology, to reveal detailed causation of metabolic function and disorder. These were critical in the development and research into steroid hormones and the human endocrine system.

The dawning of the scientific age in the 16th century lead to a more systematic cataloging of correlations between potential dangers and the corresponding remedies for human physiology—not only in the larger macro context of disorders affecting the visible anatomy, but also in the smaller microscopic level. The concurrent advances in technological engineering had by the mid-20th century pushed the field of biochemistry toward a new understanding of medical causation at the molecular level. Research into steroids and their role in human physiology played a significant role in this convergence and its research, which hitherto had been confined to the academic community, revealed itself to the broader society through a host of new and effective chemical-based treatments available directly to the consumer. The introduction of the first oral contraceptive in 1960 is one of many examples of new solutions to old problems seemingly easily achieved through a simple pill.

STEROIDS, SYNTHETICS, AND THE BIOCHEMICAL REVOLUTION

When it began, the specific research into steroids did not hold out much promise for health and medicine. The pursuit was more chemical than medical, and it rarely extended outside the laboratory. It was not until 1936 that researchers fully recognized the common molecular structure of steroid hormones, and that was only due to recent work in stereochemistry and its meaning on biochemical function. Yet, the actual start of specific research into steroids as a unique source for chemical-based metabolism began much earlier.

HISTORY OF A WORD

The word *steroid* was not specifically coined until 1936, after chemists had identified, isolated, and characterized many hormones that shared the same molecular shape (gonane), and they began to group them together under the new umbrella term. The word was derived from the word *sterol* by adding the Greek suffix *oeides*, which means "of like kind" and is simplified as "-oid."

Hormones

The real story began in 1905 when the London professor, Ernest Starling, gave a series of lectures that described a system of communication between organs orchestrated through chemical reactions. During his speech, he first coined the word "hormone" to describe those "chemical messengers" who sped "from cell to cell along the bloodstream" to coordinate the various parts throughout the body. Perhaps, it was the power of giving a specific name to an idea that had only existed as an intriguing possibility for explaining human physiology that really launched the search for steroids. Previous researchers in Germany and France had hinted at the idea of such chemical-based communication systems, but Starling named the vehicle by which the communication occurred.

Starling's introduction of the term "hormone" also happened to coincide with another breakthrough in the study of bile acids. For years, chemists tried to unlock the purpose behind the digestive fluids that seem to be found in a variety of animals and humans alike. Cholesterol had been discovered in the early 1800s, but it was viewed simply as a kind of digestive fluid found in gall stones and, recently, discovered in the blood (the word was derived from the Greek *cholé*, meaning bile or gall). By the turn of the 1900s, chemists noted a chemical relationship between cholesterol and choleic acids, in so far as none of them were soluble in water, but all were fat soluble. This discovery prompted scientists to search for a deeper, molecular commonality between them. Starling's description of hormones that travelled throughout the body as chemical messengers placed an entirely new light on the role of cholesterol as something more significant than a digestive acid, launching the path to steroid research.

For the next 20 years, chemists began to examine more closely the chemical relationships between internal organs. Most research effort was focused on identifying and isolating the characteristics of specific hormones that were related to particular organs. In 1926, Charles Harington was the first chemist to identify and synthesize thyroxine—which is a nonsteroid protein hormone produced by the thyroid. The following year, Heinrich Wieland and Adolf Windaus successfully isolated and identified the molecular construction of cholesterol, which confirmed the connection between it and other bile acids that had by that time become known collectively as sterols, and they were found in human and animals and plants alike.

The interspecies relationship was discovered a decade earlier by Friedrich Gudernatsch, who used tissues from the thyroid of a horse to stimulate frogs into maturation directly from tadpole. The realization that hormones could be derived from any number of plants and animals and still, in theory, maintain their active nature in other animals—and possibly in humans—was a major incentive for further research. Wieland's and Windhaus's identification of the common molecular structure accelerated the pace of hormone research. Between the years 1929 and 1936, the molecular structure of estrane, androsterone, progesterone, and vitamin D were identified, characterized, and synthesized. By 1936, their common molecular relationship was understood beyond that initially theorized by Wieland and Windhaus, and these hormones finally became more commonly known as steroids.

First Marketable Steroid: Cortisone

Just prior to the Second World War, a doctor at the Mayo clinic specializing in rheumatoid arthritis cases noticed a trend among patients who found relief under certain unexpected (and seemingly unrelated) conditions—pregnancy, jaundice, and during postsurgery recovery. Dr. Philip Hench theorized there was some special substance X that was responsible for the changes and set about looking for it. In early 1941, Hench contacted Professor Edward Kendall to discuss possible options, and they both agreed to try one of the new steroids that Kendall had isolated from the adrenal cortex. Unfortunately, the process of isolating and synthesizing steroid hormones required a great deal of resources. For example, in 1934, Adolf Butenandt used the ovaries of 50,000 sows to produce just 20 milligrams of progesterone—about four teaspoons worth of chemical. Similarly, in 1938, when Edward Kendall first isolated cortisol, he required the adrenal glands of 20,000 cattle. In late 1941, United States entered the war and during that time of resource scarcity it took seven years for Kendall to synthesize enough cortisone for Hench to use on his rheumatoid arthritis patients. Nevertheless, the positive results were recognized almost immediately.

Cortisone was the first steroid to be used as a therapeutic treatment. Rheumatoid arthritis was a painful and often debilitating disease which had, up to that point, no known remedies. The discovery that cortisone might aid in relief created instant demand among the medical community and industrialists. Kendall received support from Merck and Company to research alternate methods for synthesis. Based on Gudernatsch's discovery that hormones could be derived from almost any living material, Kendall researched analogues in the plant kingdom and discovered the African Strophanthus plant as the starting material for creating a synthetic form of cortisone. Merck marketed the drug in 1949, and the following year the Nobel Prize committee recognized both Kendall and Hensch for their work.

Steroids and the Chemical Revolution

Commercial success from cortisone motivated researchers in a variety of disciplines (botany, biology, and chemistry) to explore potential sources for synthesizing chemical analogues of known hormones. It was at this time that Djerassi worked with Russell Marker to find a synthesis for progesterone from Mexican yams. That discovery not only launched Djerassi's later career as the "Father of the Pill," but it also resuscitated a flagging Mexican agricultural economy as the demand for yams increased significantly. Scientists used a saponin steroid extracted from the yams, diosgenin to synthesize progesterone, testosterone, and cortisone. The cooperative relationship between chemists and a new emerging pharmaceutical industry stimulated research in dozens of related fields.

Once scientists were able to more easily gain access to purified forms of steroid hormones, then they could more specifically study the complicated processes of the endocrine system from the level of molecular interaction. Of greatest interest during the 1950s were the cascading reactions and feedback loops between various hormones and their related releasing factors. New resources meant more sophisticated technologies, and researchers delved ever deeper into the microcosm of cellular construction and chromosomal activity. Of particular utility was the new **tracer techniques** used to track the changes in molecular structure after synthesis. By the 1960s, computer models were used to determine the molecular structure of substances that may not even exist in natural form.

The relative flexibility of the steroidal gonane structure allows chemists to change and alter associated substituents without undermining the basic function of the molecule. As intellectual and technological innovations combined with the increasing industrial resources, medical research became much more aggressive. Scientists not only discovered new steroid hormones to reveal previously unknown interactions within the endocrine system, but they also customized synthetic steroid hormones to enhance certain positive properties while diminishing other less desirable traits. This revolution in biochemistry largely began with steroid research, but it was not limited to hormone. Other medical specialties, including fields in psychiatry, also partnered with the increasing resources of the pharmaceutical companies to reexamine their procedures beginning with an understanding of the smallest operations.

Today, researchers study the smallest operations of DNA transcription and other subcellular activity. Instead of categorically identifying and isolating hormones, modern researchers strive to isolate specific expressions of each gene with the eventual objective of manipulating the mechanisms that activate or inhibit their function. Creating specific molecules to control substrates or receptors for particular enzymes, hormones and neurotransmitters are called **rational design**.

Complete rational design is still an unachieved goal. It is like a giant, immensely complex remote control system, and doctors hope to identify the buttons that activate certain functions in the human body. Unfortunately, the remote is still far too large for researchers to fully understand what and where each button might be. More significantly, the buttons invariably activate multiple functions, and scientists are left trying new combinations and sequences to isolate the functions they most desire. Nevertheless, by the 1970s, computers, nuclear magnetic resonance imaging, and high-pressure liquid chromatography brought the dream of rational design closer to reality. Advances in cardiovascular drugs, calcium blockers, ACE inhibitors, cholesterol reduction, antihistamines, anti-inflammatories, and a host of other chemicals increase a physician's reliance on drug-based therapies as their most common treatment option. Throughout this era of discovery, policymakers and the general public alike both encouraged the scientific community to increase the rate of new innovation, and also reacted strongly when certain combinations had unwanted social consequences.

PILLS, DRUGS, AND THE CHEMICAL CULTURE

The postwar 1950s experienced a degree of cultural consensus that was influenced by twin developments in academia and industry. The Second World War inspired unprecedented levels of scientific development, especially in the areas of physics, mechanical engineering, and other fields related to weaponry, transportation, communication, and logistical support. In the field of medicine, significant achievements emerged in treating traumatic injuries and infections typically associated with the battlefield. Blood transfusion, skin grafts, and gas masks join penicillin as some of the era's most significant inventions. Like many other chemical compounds of the time, penicillin was discovered and isolated prior to the war (by Alexander Fleming in 1928), but it took the exigencies of wartime demands to equip Ernst Chain and Howard Florey with the resources necessary to discover mass production. Their success is credited with saving thousands of lives by preventing secondary infections suffered during the traumatic casualties of the D-Day invasion in 1944—and all three men shared a Nobel Prize after the war ended in 1945.

The pace of scientific innovation did not slacken following the war. Instead, the research objectives shifted from military to nonmilitary purposes, though the government maintained a significant presence in both research and development. The nature of American industry shifted from producing goods to producing services, with the balance formally tipping to the latter after 1956. A growing demand for white-collar jobs encouraged scientific exploration, and a thriving economy encouraged investment. The gross national product increased from $200 billion to $300 billion during the 1940s, but it nearly doubled to $500 billion by 1960. This hyperactive economic environment created a marketplace that was eager for new discoveries, and the pharmaceutical industry fell easily in place.

Pharmaceutical Industrial Complex

During the 1950s, drug companies experienced a sort of golden age as a new relationship emerged between academic researchers working at universities, pharmaceutical companies funding (and marketing) their discoveries, and medical schools and hospitals becoming increasingly dependent on the new drugs for practical implementation. Often, biochemists might operate in all three realms. Major drug companies like Merck, Pfizer, Parke-Davis, and Smith, Kline & French all offered incentives, jobs, and even shares in partnership with research professors, as did their smaller companies. For example, Carl Djerassi worked at Stanford University and conducted research for Syntex Laboratories as an employee. After discovering the contraceptive potential of his progesterone synthesis, Djerassi brokered his valuable patent into a presidency of the company. The positive side of this relationship was that the delay between discovery and public availability (often called a **drug lag**) was significantly reduced. Many drugs that were initially isolated and characterized in the 1920s and 1930s were patented, marketed, and mass produced in the 1950s and others were being researched for their immediate practical applications. The negative side of this industrial complex is that there may be conflicts of interest between researchers and marketing. Academic scientists were encouraged to follow paths of discovery that fulfilled economic demand and they could be tempted to overlook (or ignore) potential dangers when such revelations might impact the marketing of the drug.

Public reaction to this academic-industrial complex emerged as early as the 1950s. In one example, the Parke-Davis pharmaceutical company had advertised its synthesis of chloromycetin as completely nontoxic, and yet it lead to the deaths of several children whose physiological profile triggered aplastic anemia. Lawsuits charged gross negligence and false advertising on the part of the drug company, and later evidence suggested that the company did indeed soft peddle the side effects in order to encourage doctor's prescriptions. Perhaps, most shocking to the public, however, were the epidemic of birth defects associated with the use of **thalidomide**. A German pharmaceutical company, Grünental, developed and obtained a patent on the synthesis in 1954 and within three years marketed the drug under the name Tholimid. It was the first nonbarbiturate-based sedative, which meant it was not habit forming and it was advertised as completely safe for everyone, including pregnant women (initial tests suggested that the drug would not be able to pass through the placental barrier). This new "wonder drug" was sold in countries around the world, with sales that rivaled that of aspirin (the previous "wonder drug" from the 1910s). In 1960, Australian doctor William McBride began prescribing the drug as a cure for morning sickness, which was a practice imitated worldwide, even though the drug was not intended for that purpose. Almost immediately, McBride noticed the sudden increase in a rare birth defect called phocomelia, which inhibits the development and formation of limbs resulting in shortened or absent arms or legs that ended in flipper like hands extending off the trunk of the body. McBride and German pediatrician Widukind Lenz are credited with identifying and later proving the association between thalidomide and phocomelia. The connection was not obvious at first because the drug manufacturer had indicated that it bore no harmful side effects and most mothers using the drug gave birth to healthy children. Indeed, later research revealed that it was only one optical substituent of thalidomide that caused the inhibited development. Nevertheless, there were at least 10,000 cases of phocomelia reported in 46 countries before it was banned worldwide in 1962.

The United States avoided these birth defects because the FDA had held off approving the drug until further tests could be made. The main concern of the delegated FDA reviewer, Frances Kelsey, was that it might lead to irreversible peripheral neuropathy but there was not enough clinical information to be certain. During the 1950s, the drug companies did not need FDA approval before beginning clinical trials and the tests did not often follow uniform procedures. In the case of thalidomide, the American drug company Richardson Merrell tested the drug (which they labeled Kevadon) by sending 2.5 million tablets out to a 1,000 doctors treating 20,000 patients, which included 3,760 women of childbearing age—a little more than 200 were pregnant at the time. Very few doctors reported their findings and Richardson Merrell had very little documentation to offer Frances Kelsey to prove the drug's safety or effectiveness. After the discovery of the phocomelia connection became known worldwide, President John Kennedy heralded Kelsey's hesitation in approving the drug in the United States and awarded her the President's Award for Distinguished Federal Service. He used the incident to push for more stringent FDA regulations to tighten and track preclinical and clinical testing for all new pharmaceuticals, leading Congress to approve the Food, Drug and Cosmetic Act of 1962. The new legislation doubled and often tripled the average drug lag time out to 8–12 years between discovery and implementation, but American public strongly approved the new policy.

Tranquilizers and the Baby Boom

The public's growing concern of the medical community's seemingly heavy-handed embrace of chemical solutions was reinforced by another trend in American culture that had little to do with science. In addition to a booming activity in industry and research, the postwar generation experienced a boom in new children. The number of new births increased nearly 25 percent in 1946 over the previous year, from 2.8 million to 3.5 million, and this rate of population growth remained constant for more than a decade afterward. This baby boom resulted in an explosion in the number of families with young children, and the earliest of the new youngsters did not reach adulthood until early 1960s. As a result, the 1950s cultural priorities focused primarily on the needs of young parents and their growing children. Health, education, and community were popular concerns. By the mid-1960s, as the new generation reached an age where they began making their own purchasing decisions, advertisers shifted their marketing campaigns toward younger audiences. The cultural priorities also shifted, though not without some contest from the older generations.

For the mainstream of American public, recreational drug use in the 1950s was mostly limited to alcohol, caffeine, and tobacco. There was, however, a growing dependence and use of psychotropic (mood altering) drugs for therapeutic purposes among young adults. In 1955, Wallace Laboratories introduced its synthesis of meprobamate under the trade name Miltown (named after the town in which it was manufactured, Milltown, New Jersey). Frank Berger and Bernard Ludwig had first isolated and synthesized the drug only five years earlier from mephenesin, which was originally used to preserve penicillin. Berger noticed the tranquilizing effect of mephenesin and published his findings in 1946. He and Ludwig searched for an analogue compound that isolated the tranquilizing properties from its other toxic side effects. Miltown became an instant success because it induced many of the same effects as opiate derivatives, but in a milder form and without the negative reputation.

Narcotics had been known and abused since the 19th century, and through the evidence of history and experience, the public strongly associated heroine, morphine, and marijuana with addiction and vice. Yet, Miltown was a new synthetic analogue sold in a simple pill form (not smoked, injected, or inhaled), which offered a sort of legitimacy to the objective of emotional sedation. Following the war, especially, doctors and psychiatrists noted an increase in generalized anxiety, which is a sense of fear or turmoil rising with no particular cause. Miltown was marketed as a mild tranquilizer that could be prescribed for generalized anxiety during the normal course of an otherwise healthy lifestyle and it was an instant success. Within two years, its manufacturer, Carter Medicine Company, was selling more than a billion tablets a year. Miltown was the bestselling drug ever marketed in the United States, claiming more than a third of all prescriptions during the late 1950s. More than one out of every seven adults used it with some regularity. As the historian Andrea Tone describes it, Miltown was viewed by ordinary healthy Americans as a sort of emotional aspirin and there were few negative sentiments associated with it.

Fears of Recreational Drug Use

The popularity of tranquilizers for therapeutic use does not mean that the 1950s mainstream approved of the recreational use of drugs. A growing literary movement in America, known as the Beat Generation, included poets and writers who wrote about casual sex and drug use, but they were initially received with trepidation and remained a marginal fringe of American artists. Other older and more reputable authors, such as Aldous Huxley, also began writing about the virtues of hallucinogenic (**psychedelic**) drugs such as peyote and psilocybin mushrooms, but these were not widely known. Younger beat writers like Jack Kerouac, Allen Ginsberg, and William Burroughs wrote about their experiences with recreational drug use, but their works were frequently banned or censored by the mainstream adults who had little sympathy for their activity. The parents of young children were concerned by these depictions and rejected such drug abuse. Yet, these harsh reactions changed during the 1960s as those young children, the first members of the baby boom generation, began to come of age. The beat generation was far more fully embraced by the emerging youth of the 1960s than they ever had been by the adults of the 1950s.

One of the most notable signs of cultural clash occurred when Harvard professor Timothy Leary began publicly advocating the use of psychedelic drugs as a means for achieving higher consciousness. He became most associated with the use of **lysergic acid diethylamide**, more commonly known as LSD (or simply acid). The compound was originally isolated and synthesized in 1938 by Albert Hofmann, which he derived from ergotamine. Its hallucinogenic properties were discovered by accident five years later, and were capitalized on after the war as a potential tool for combating schizophrenia. Sandoz Laboratories marketed the drug under the name Delysid in 1947. LSD was not the first synthesis of a hallucinogenic. Ernst Späth synthesized the active ingredient in peyote and Mescaline, which was used later in the 1950s research of psychiatrist Humphrey Osmand. Similarly, phenocyclidine (commonly known as PCP) was synthesized in 1926 before being patented and marketed under the name

Sernyl by Parke-Davis as an antipsychotic. Albert Hofman later synthe-sized the active ingredient in psilocybin mushrooms in 1958, though they were never marketed. What made LSD unique was that a seemingly cred-ible academic researcher, Leary, promoted the drug as a pathway to higher spiritual fulfillment.

Leary personally experimented with hallucinogenic drugs during the late 1950s, and he received a grant to study the effect of LSD on the re-habilitation of released prisoners in 1960 while serving as a lecturer at Harvard. The study, known as the Concord Prison Experiment, drew the attention of beat poet Allen Ginsberg and other popular cultural figures. Leary interpreted the study results to indicate strong support for LSD as a tool in reducing criminal recidivism. These findings were later refuted, but Leary still used this study as a platform for promoting LSD as a non-addictive alternative to alcohol and as a means for escaping the bonds of natural perception leading to emotional, psychological, and even spiritual fulfillment. Harvard University fired Leary for his outspoken declarations, but the publicity gained him a large following of supporters among young college students who were already experimenting with individual freedom and new adulthood.

Legal Prohibitions against New Chemicals

During the 1950s and most of the 1960s, LSD, PCP, mescaline, and other new synthesis of hallucinogenic drugs were legal under existing fed-eral and state laws. Marijuana was illegal, but LSD could be freely used with no consequences. With the help of supporters, Leary set up a large house in 1962 where he based his International Foundation for Internal Freedom. He invited college students and celebrities to come and experi-ence LSD for the purpose of higher enlightenment. The negative public reaction among mainstream adults was fierce, and by mid-decade a move-ment arose seeking the ban of LSD and similar drugs resulting in various states passing laws prohibiting its use for any purpose (therapeutic or oth-erwise). In 1966, Leary started the League of Spiritual Discovery, which he described as a new religion that held LSD as its holy sacrament. This was an attempt to use freedom of religion to sidestep the inevitable federal prohibitions. He and his supporters toured college campuses in 1967 and distributed pamphlets titled "Start your own religion." Despite these ef-forts, Federal prohibition came in 1967, and Leary faced a series of legal troubles for the next decade which led to his incarceration several times.

The actual use of hallucinogenic remained very small to the relative proportion of the population. No statistics are available for the 1960s, but when the government began compiling such statistics in the 1970s, the numbers reflect relatively low usage. Among adults, 26 years or older in 1974 (which meant they were in their college years during the mid-1960s), only 1.3 percent had ever used hallucinogenic drugs. That number was higher (16%) for young adults aged 18–25, though most of these would have been still in their preteens during the early 1960s, suggesting that their usage dated from the later 1960s and early 1970s. The number of young adults currently using the drug fell to 2.5 percent. Nevertheless, the public sensationalism of Leary and his group of young followers had an impact on other drugs, particularly marijuana. The number of young adults who had ever tried marijuana in 1974 grew from less than 4 percent to more than 50 percent; though again, other statistics suggest that most of that experimentation began in the late 1960s and early 1970s.

Though actual drug use may have been otherwise, the popular expectation that young people were routinely experimenting with synthetic drugs of any sort for recreational use grew to the point that it became a national priority among politicians in the early 1970s. President Richard Nixon pointed to rising crime rates and associated increase in drug use as a significant issue in his "Law and Order" platform. In 1970, with Nixon's strong support, the Congress passed the Comprehensive Drug Abuse and Control Act, which required pharmaceutical companies, hospitals, and doctors to take specific steps to safeguard the physical security of their drugs and keep strict record keeping of their distribution and usage. The law reclassified all drugs into five main categories called **schedules**. Classification was based on the drug's recognized potential for abuse, its accepted therapeutic value for medical use, and its relative safety under medical supervision. At one end of the spectrum, Schedule I drugs included those that have least therapeutic value and showed high dangers for medical harm and abuse. At the other end, Schedule V drugs showed the greatest therapeutic value with the least associated risks of harm or abuse. Three years later, shortly after his second term victory, Nixon issued an executive order creating the Drug Enforcement Agency, which was a single consolidated body responsible for the enforcement of federal drug laws.

Clearly, the therapeutic use of steroids played little role in the public rising fear of epidemic drug abuse. Nevertheless, the initial research into steroid hormones contributed significantly to the direction of biochemical research, and aided in the academic-industrial complex that led to the public's new consciousness of a rising chemical culture. Moreover, even though the therapeutic use of catabolic steroids remains relatively less controversial than its anabolic cousins, both forms fall subject to the increasing oversight and regulations of the federal drug laws.

CONCLUSION

The Hippocratic Oath was first written down more than 2,500 years ago. Though numerous versions and translations have been used through the years, the classical version begins the list of principles governing patient care with the pledge "I will keep them from harm." In the same spirit, the Federal Drug Abuse and Control Act classified chemicals according to whether they offer any therapeutic aid and whether they might be abused, possibly causing harm to themselves or others. At the level of direct patient interaction, doctors historically weigh the benefits of a given treatment against the possible dangers. Usually, the patient is included in this decision-making process, and the doctor uses both technical knowledge and experience to make appropriate counsels. Nevertheless, it is possible that communication, either on the part of the doctor or the drug manufacturer, may limit the extent to which patients are able to make informed decisions. Governmental regulations at state and federal levels attempt to establish procedures to safeguard against these gaps, but they are imperfect. In the end, the patient is ultimately responsible for making decisions that help ensure no harm comes.

Changing Definitions

Other factors influence the decision-making process when individuals weigh therapeutic treatment options, especially as they change the definition of what constitutes harm and benefit. In traditional medicine, these terms are defined according to how a treatment might impact specific physiological functions in the body. As the scientific community gains an ever-deeper understanding of these functions—even down to the microscopic level—then assessment of harm and benefit includes more precise and more detailed explanations. At the same time, however, molecular biology is incomplete and the full knowledge of potential side effects remains elusive, especially for reactions that may take years to develop, such as cancer. The rare incidents of scandal or new revelations of hitherto unrealized side effects all served to undermine some level of authority held by the scientific researchers. When coupled with other sociopolitical concerns about conflicts of interest between academia and industry, the potential for distrust compounds. In part, this may explain some of the attraction of nontraditional approaches to medicine that use alternative standards for measuring help or harm.

In addition, the cultural environment since the 1960s has contributed to a significant reliance on biochemistry to solve medical problems. This chemical culture may have numerous implications in society, especially in terms of defining social expectations and potential costs. Like the progressives of the early part of the century, the postwar biochemical revolution encourages confidence among researchers to uncover and resolve almost any disorder, if given enough time, talent, and resources. The pursuit of synthetic drugs developed through rational design may produce an unintended side effect of intolerance and impatience among the consuming public. Disorders such as mild generalized anxiety, which may affect virtually anyone at any time, may have been ignored or simply endured in ages past, but now require proactive treatment. Other milder symptoms such as headaches, coughing, sleepiness, or fatigue might traditionally have been dealt with simple rest. Now, the average consumer often searches for a chemical compound to relieve suffering rather than tolerate even momentary discomfort. Such changes in the expectation of good health can impact individual choices as to whether they deem the immediate relief of short-term symptoms as important as the potential long-term dangers of more complicated treatments.

Scientific Probabilities

There are also philosophical implications of an increasing reliance on chemical therapies. What if the cause of a particular ailment cannot be discovered? Or what if the cause is known and yet a cure remains undiscovered? How does that impact anxiety levels in an age where science holds such optimism for almost unending solutions? How does such incomplete knowledge impact individual decision making for long-term health care strategies?

PROBABILITY AND ELECTIVE THERAPY

In 2013, actress Angelina Jolie voluntarily underwent radical double mastectomy at the age of 37. The procedure removed the tissues of both breasts as a prophylactic measure and not because any sign of the disease had yet appeared. Jolie had a family history of breast cancer and she carried a mutation of the BRCA1 gene, which increased her probability of developing cancer to 87 percent with a 50 percent risk of developing ovarian cancer. There was no certainty of contracting the disease, and many women may live with the same genetic mutation without being affected. The American Cancer Society indicates that the potential for surviving breast and ovarian cancer for five years or more, after early detection, is more than 90 percent. Yet, the price of surgery seemed less problematic than the risk of diagnosis. Through a series of surgical procedures, the physical structure of the breasts could be maintained largely intact, while the underlying tissue was

> removed. Some women decide that the potential future risks outweighed the costs and risks of the surgery, and elected to have the procedure. Yet, questions remain about whether the removal of the breast tissue from a healthy woman may lead to unknown risks in the future. Most studies involve subjects who also suffer from concurrent diseases like cancer. Very little research exists on the impact of mastectomy on the endocrine system of an otherwise healthy woman.

Other observers may question whether health care decisions should be based on potential rather than actualized risks. These kinds of issues are equally relevant for other kinds of disorders. As the health care community increases its knowledge of internal systems, including the complicated reactions of the endocrine system, then the potential for decisions based on probabilities increases. Particular concerns are raised when funding and health insurance is involved. Certain governmental agencies and other health insurance bodies base their decisions for authorizing certain treatments on the probability of likely success rather than on the actual circumstances of the individual. When resources are scarce, there is legitimate concern that some people may be unfairly discriminated because their biological profile suggests potential dangers in the future. Strong criticisms from both sides of the political aisle raise questions about overly relying on scientific probability when making individual health care decisions. These and other related questions illustrate the importance of policy and political decision making as related to the availability of certain therapeutic options.

Elective Treatment and Pursuit of Perfection

As science and technology reveal an ever-increasing array of solutions for both actual and potential disorders, individual decision making may gradually veer away from questions that focus exclusively on health needs and begin to include questions related to comfort or preference. Deciding whether to have major surgery to avoid a potentially life-threatening disease certainly falls under the realm of health needs. Yet, decisions about whether or not to take certain chemical supplements in order to run faster, or work longer, or look stronger are based on preferences and not need. To some extent, these issues are less commonly associated with catabolic steroids, which are almost exclusively used for therapeutic treatments. But they play a major role in decisions related to anabolic steroid use. Decisions to using biochemistry to achieve the perfect body, or to gain competitive advantage, or to hold back the powers of age have deep social, political, and philosophical implications. The history of this side of steroid research is covered more thoroughly in the next chapter.

CHAPTER 3

Historical Background of Performance-Enhancing Steroids

As World War II came to a close, Paul de Kruif published a popularized discussion of testosterone in *The Male Hormone*. In it, he recounts the discovery of testosterone and his personal experience with taking the hormone as a dietary supplement. After a year of daily doses, the 55-year-old noticed significant improvements in his muscle development as well as a general increase in energy levels. He described the effects of testosterone as if it were a special elixir used by "the human body to be able to build the very stuff of its own life." The book envisioned a future where testosterone would overcome the natural decline of age and extend the range of man's natural vitality.

Kruif was a former microbiologist turned science writer, who first gained fame in 1926 for his dramatic portraits of early endocrinologists in *Microbe Hunters*. He was physically large and imposing, and was known as a colorful storyteller who made scientific discovery interesting to the general public. The narrative tone of the testosterone story and Kruif's explanation of its virtues painted an optimistic view of its future role in medicine. Testosterone made him feel like a younger, stronger, more virulent man. It was the key to manliness and a key to youth—all young men naturally produce testosterone of their own in abundance, but as old age sets in, time eventually steals it away. Kruif knew he was reliving his youth through artificial means, but as he promised, "I will try to renew my aging tissues with testosterone as long as I can." Though he initially feared the contemptuous smiles of those who doubted the power of the hormone,

Kruif admitted, "I'm no longer ashamed that it's no longer made to its old degree by my old, aging body. . . . It's chemical crutches. It's borrowed manhood. It's borrowed time. But just the same, it's what makes bulls bulls."

Perhaps, Kruif's depiction of testosterone's importance was somewhat glamorized for the sake his book, but it nevertheless reflected a popular view of the time. Unlike the catabolic steroid hormones that were pursued in an effort to fill the gaps of understanding in emerging fields of biochemistry and endocrinology, the anabolic steroids (testosterone, in particular) were studied first for their potential as a source for increasing male vitality. Scientists, both then and now, can be found who describe anabolic steroids as a key to delaying the effects of old age—something akin to finding the fountain of youth. It was not until the biochemical revolution of the 1950s that anabolic steroids became more associated with its other practical application of competitive enhancement. Once that association took root, the characterization (and reputation) of anabolic steroids changed dramatically. Nevertheless, as late as the 1960s, anabolic steroids were often viewed more as helpful dietary supplements (like vitamins) than they were as chemical means for competitive dishonesty.

The effects of anabolic steroids on performance spread by word of mouth among athletes very quickly after the first commercial synthetic anabolic steroid was introduced. Public awareness, however, was much slower to follow. During the 1960s and 1970s, as recreational drug use began to attract public notice, and as mainstream society became more sensitive to the harmful consequence of drug use in general, the public reaction to ergogenic drugs gradually shifted as well. First, international amateur sports associations (including the Olympic movement) shifted from general indifference in the 1950s, to more proactive concern in the 1960s, and increasing alarm in the 1970s. Then, as the dangers of steroids and other ergogenic drugs became manifest in professional venues during the 1980s and 1990s, the fan base reactions turned strongly negative. For the sake of athletic safety and competitive fairness, professional athletic associations, sports franchises, and political legislators systematically prohibited anabolic steroid use for the purposes of performance enhancement.

THE MALE HORMONE

In some ways, the scientific path of anabolic steroids followed the same trail of research used by the more therapeutic catabolic hormones. Since the 1910s, budding endocrinologists adopted a systematic approach of isolating the secretions of each organ in an attempt to catalog hormone messengers thought to be responsible for metabolic function. Each new discovery followed the same pattern: isolate the hormone related to a particular organ; determine its characteristics and, if possible its molecular structure; and then attempt a partial synthesis as a sort of verification. Insofar as testosterone was recognized as the main hormone of the gonads, then that process echoed the procedures used for several other hormones, such as the nonsteroid hormone thyroxine (isolated from the thyroid) and the female sex hormone estrone (isolated from the ovaries).

In other ways, though, research into testosterone was often governed by a practical search for whatever substance that was responsible for those physical qualities that 19th century scientists associated with maleness. Most research concentrated on understanding the male hormone and not on anabolic steroids. Unlike cortisone, which was discovered before its therapeutic potential was recognized, the functional purpose of testosterone was precisely what drove its initial research. Further development awaited only the invention of new tools and theories of molecular biology to make testosterone available for specific research application.

Ancient Observations

The association between the testes and male secondary sex characteristics has been recognized since ancient times. More the 2,800 years ago, Assyrian officials sought to strengthen their bureaucracy by castrating the leaders of various governmental offices. The intent was not punitive—Assyrian rulers in their typically blunt manner attempted to prevent certain positions of power from being handed down as hereditary lines, and using **eunuchs** as bureaucratic officials was an effective approach. Very quickly, though, the secondary effects of castration became equally apparent. Eunuchs never fully developed in the way other men did. Nearly 400 years later, the Greek teacher Aristotle recognized that the effects of castration were similar between species, and often differed depending on whether the castration occurred as youth or as adults. Castrated adults (like the Assyrian bureaucrats), cease growing facial hair and became physically weaker with less muscle tone. Castrated boys never developed adult characteristics. They never grow pubic hair, remain physically slight in build, and maintain a high-pitched voice. Aristotle specifically identified the effect of castrating birds, "his crest grows sallow, he ceases to crow, and forgoes sexual activity." Even in ancient times, astute observers recognized that the testicles contained something that governed the outward characteristics that made men look and sound (and perhaps act) like men.

TESTES AND POWER AROUND THE WORLD

Ancient East Indian texts recommended eating animal testicles to combat impotence. This was echoed by the Central American medical practices: indigenous Mexicans made a tea made of the grounded and toasted testicles of the coatimundi (looks like a skinny raccoon), while Ecuadorian Amazonians used the ground bone of the coati penis. In South Africa, witch doctors used testicles (and other human body parts cut off while the person was still alive) to brew *muthi* potions that held magical healing powers to promote strength and confidence. In Southeast Asia, the penis and testicles of tigers were prized for their aphrodisiac properties. Such practices all reflect a primitive belief in sympathetic magic, which assumes "like produces like," and therefore eating or consuming the source of another's virility (animal or human) will transfer their virility to yourself. Their prevalence indicates an almost universal understanding that the male gonads were clearly tied to secondary male characteristics.

In an oblique way, such primitive observations reveal a grain of scientific truth. Indigenous shamans may not have understood the endocrine system, but they recognized that there was something in the tissues of male gonads—regardless of the species—that contributes to those characteristics that define maleness (although the claim of curing impotence is entirely unfounded).

Berthold and Brown-Séquard

In the mid-1800s, a French physiologist Arnold Berthold attempted to duplicate Aristotle's observations of castrated birds through a famous experiment he performed on six male chickens. Berthold castrated four of the six birds when they were still young, and using the castrated pieces, he surgically implanted the testicles in the abdomens of two of the castrated chickens. The two who were not castrated grew to be normal, aggressive roosters with adult feathers and rigid combs. The two that were castrated with no other changes, never matured as roosters, with undeveloped feathers and combs, and exhibited no aggressive behaviors typically associated with roosters. Yet, the two castrated birds that received surgical implants developed into mature adults and exhibited the same characteristics as the two that had never been castrated. As a further control, Berthold later removed the implanted testes from the abdomen of one the two birds and it quickly began to revert to the condition of the other two castrated chickens. From this experiment, Berthold recognized that since the transplanted testicles were not connected to anything else in the birds' system, then the potency of the male rooster must have come from something in the tissues of the testicle.

About 40 years after Berthold's experiment, in the late 1880s, renowned physiologist Charles Brown-Séquard presented a paper before the Biological Society in Paris on his research into the "Elixir of Life." Brown-Séquard was already recognized for extensive research on the adrenal glands, the spinal cord, and the nervous system, which resulted in more than 500 separate publications throughout his career. Like others of his time, Brown-Séquard believed that the internal organs acted together in response to some kind of chemical (the word hormone had not yet been coined) that passed through the bloodstream. As he got older, he developed a theory that the chemical was probably related to the sex organs, and that old age and senility were the natural consequences of the body ceasing to produce that vital chemical. The product of Brown-Séquard's research was an elixir derived from tissues extracted from the gonads of living animals: guinea pigs, lambs, dogs, and so on. He sedated the animals, used a syringe to extract the tissues, pulverized the materials in a mortar, mixed it with water, filtered out the visible tissues, and then reinjected it into himself.

After only a few days, the more than 70-year-old Brown-Séquard noticed he could work longer days in the lab, whereas previously he had been forced to take extended breaks every few hours. In his own words, Brown-Séquard claimed that his "nervous activity has been increased in every way. Muscular strength has become much more considerable than in the past; the intestinal and vesicle contractions have taken on a vigor which they had not had for a long time; ability to do intellectual work has been greatly increased. I have discovered, following these injections, how one regains youth." His elixir became global news, with reports reaching as far as India and San Francisco. For a time, some doctors outside the mainstream embraced his testicular-extract solution as a secret to extending life. The more conservative establishment, however, was less interested. There were more than a few reports of toxic reactions to this elixir and deaths attributed to the procedure. Moreover, Brown-Séquard himself died about five years later at the age of 77 and the elixir (with its related search for a chemical fountain of youth) was temporarily discredited—at least for a generation.

Biochemical Discovery

By the 1920s, the systematic isolation and characterization of hormone inspired a class of young researchers to reexamine Berthold and Brown-Séquard's experiments. Under the direction of University of Chicago professor Fred Koch, a 23-year-old graduate assistant student Lemuel McGee based his doctoral dissertation on Berthold's rooster experiments. Instead of using the testes extracted from the chickens, McGee used 40 pounds of bull testes, from which he managed to extract just 20 milligrams of material. At that point, the gonad material had been unidentified and McGee injected it into castrated chickens numerous times, successfully repeating Berthold's original study. The use of cross-species gonad material, not only affirmed Berthold, but also lent some credence to Brown-Séquard's initial observations that there was a common vitality found in male gonads of all mammals.

Almost immediately, researchers in half a dozen separate labs began focusing on how to isolate the material that could reverse the effects of castration—the object of their research was called simply "the male hormone". Some researchers hypothesized that since hormones travelled through the bloodstream, then it was likely processed through the liver. Shortly thereafter, Casimir Funk (who first formulated the idea of vitamins) and his research assistant Benjamin Harrow from the City College of New York discovered that they could achieve similar results in castrated roosters without physically extracting it from male gonads—they extracted it instead from male urine. Following this discovery, another grad student at the University of Rochester, Charles Kochakian, was given $500 to collect thousands of gallons of urine from his fellow medical students to study whether the male hormone of humans could energize the metabolism of a castrated dog. The study initially proved ineffective, but Kochakian continued the research undaunted.

By the early 1930s, the pharmaceutical industry joined the effort to cost effectively isolate the male hormone (and then begin marketing it in some way). Major companies in the Netherlands, Germany, and Switzerland invested considerable research money into the project and a race began among the researchers to correctly identify the compound and its molecular structure. Within a week of each other, the German Adolf Butenandt and the Swiss Leopold Ruzicka independently published accounts of how they synthesized the male hormone from cholesterol. They named it after the male gonad from which it originated—testosterone—, and later earned a Noble Prize for their discovery. The following year, Kochakian and his advisor John Murlin successfully isolated the anabolic characteristics of testosterone in 1936.

Eugenics and the Elixir of Life

Perhaps more than any other steroid hormone at that time, the discovery, isolation, and identification of testosterone captured the imagination of the scientific community. Kochakian and Murlin uncovered both anabolic and androgenic characteristics of testosterone—the steroid not only contributed to increases in metabolic energy leading to muscle growth, but it also increased secondary sex characteristics, with wide ranging and diverse results among the various animal species. In 1938, in the year prior to the outbreak of war in Europe, there were major conferences in New York and Sweden that focused primarily on the question of how to separate the anabolic characteristics from testosterone's androgenic traits. Human testing of testosterone began almost immediately, but during the war, the published accounts dealt primarily with its therapeutic uses, particularly in the replenishing of negative nitrogen balances among starving men.

During the war years, much of the scientific research was restricted. Later historians have hypothesized that since Butenandt and his research lab that first synthesized testosterone was in Germany, then German researchers must have undertaken more extensive experiments of testosterone's anabolic effects on their elite storm troopers—even Hitler himself has been described as an experiment subject. Therefore, by the war's end in 1945, these historians further concluded that some analogue of testosterone was already known among non-Western governments, and was in use for international sports competitions.

There is no reliable evidence that Nazi troops used anabolic steroids, but the historical rumor is popular because it coincides with the larger impression left by Nazi propaganda that they would stop at nothing, leave no scientific option unused, to create and develop a more perfect human specimen (and fighting machine.) Indeed, there is some truth in the generalization, insofar as it reflects the very real environment of a eugenics culture that heavily influenced academics during the decades prior to the war. The eugenics argument rested on a firm belief that the proper control of breeding would help ensure a stronger human stock. When set in an era where several modern governments, including the technically advanced Germans, publicly advocated eugenics programs to protect its national culture and the racial supremacy of its people, then it may be easier to understand how a certain degree of nationalist pride seeped into the realm of academic research. The discovery of testosterone, as the ultimate male hormone, was in some quarters viewed as much for its potential for creating a new *überman*—in others, it was seen more soberly as a pathway to extended life. It was in this context that Paul de Kruif echoed Brown-Séquard's dream of an elixir of life, and proclaimed that testosterone was "a new gleam of hope for prolonging man's prime of life."

EUGENICS MOVEMENT IN THE UNITED STATES

Beginning around the turn of the century in the United States, Dr. Harry Sharp of the Indiana State prison systematically operated to remove the reproductive power of inmates who he deemed to be incorrigible. He did not castrate them, but Sharp performed hundreds of vasectomies—some with patient consent and many more without. Legislatures in half the states in the country passed laws that upheld Sharp's actions and doctors in 24 states began sterilizing selected inmates at prisons and mental health facilities. When the family of one of these sterilized inmates, Carrie Buck, sued in protest, the U.S. Supreme Court affirmed the state laws. In the 1927 *Buck v. Bell* decision, Justice Oliver Wendell Holmes explained, "Three generations of imbeciles are enough." The confidence by which the academic community believed they could genetically improve the human species resulted in explicit legal action, and was not unique to the United States.

A PARALLEL HISTORY OF ERGOGENIC AIDS IN COMPETITIVE SPORTS

Despite its association with male vitality, testosterone and its related anabolic androgenic steroid analogues were not initially associated with sports and the promise of a competitive edge. That connection emerged later, after the biochemical revolution of the 1950s thrust the potential of customized metabolism into the operational game plans of amateur and professional sports authorities. Yet, even after athletes and trainers began to exploit the anabolic nature of steroid hormones, it was some time before they were seen as anything more harmful than a supercharged dietary supplement (or vitamin).

Doping and Professional Gambling

Testosterone may not have been immediately recognized as an ergogenic tool, but the practice of using some kind of chemical to alter the outcome of a sporting event was well understood long before the 20th century. The term **dope** originated from the Dutch *doop*, which the settlers in South Africa used to describe the practice of Zulu Warriors who drank an alcohol-based mixture to prepare themselves before battle. The word migrated to England where it was applied to the illegal practice of feeding various concoctions to racehorses before competition. Just as horse races were liable to be fixed, so too were the races with humans. Whenever gambling is involved, the likelihood of tampering with the competition increases, and allegations that professional athletes were being doped to improve performance became widespread. By the mid-19th century, allegations of corruption and doping grew hand in hand as professional sports emerged in England and Europe as a viable new industry.

By the late 1800s, allegations of doping were frequent enough among professional sports that observers began to distinguish between amateurs and professionals based on their commitment to the purity of the game. A professional boxer, for example, fought for the money, and if there was more money involved in throwing the fight than in winning it, then it was a rare boxer who resisted the temptation. By contrast, the amateur athlete was seen to be motivated by the thrill of competition alone, because no money was involved. For this reason, the "father of the Olympic movement," 33-year-old Pierre de Coubertin, insisted that only amateur athletes compete. Coubertin viewed sport and the Olympic movement as a pathway to strong character development, which in turn could promote peace among all nations. Amateur athletes were supposed to be beyond the temptations of gambling, doping, or unfair advantage. Similarly, the Olympic movement was intended to be pure competitive sport, without the taint of money.

First Dope: Stimulants

Coubertin's vision was a little quixotic. Amateur racers were often as driven to find some advantage to win gold as any professional might be to win the purse. Nevertheless, the presumption of nobility among amateur athletics persisted and the **International Olympic Committee** (IOC) did not specifically address the problem of doping until the 1950s, and did not have any meaningful mechanism for enforcement until the late 1960s. The late attention, though, does not mean that ergogenic drug use was not evident in previous Olympiads. During the 1904 Olympics in St. Louis, distance runner Thomas Hicks collapsed immediately after crossing the finish line to win the race and it took his trainers nearly an hour before he could be revived. Officials blamed the heat and humidity—it was a hot afternoon with temperatures in the 90s, and it is true that Hicks lost 10 pounds due to dehydration. But most inside observers (including Hick's own account) attributed the breakdown to the liquid mixture of raw eggs, brandy, and strychnine that he took three times during the last 10 miles of the race. His trainers refused to give him water because they thought it would slow him down, so they gave him the stimulant mixture instead. At that time, such mixtures were not uncommon and many trainers developed their own recipes, which they kept secret from prying eyes, in order to stimulate and get their athletes moving.

The public distinguished between the motivations of doping animals in horse or dog races and the motivations behind using chemical concoctions to stimulate the human athlete. The animal had no choice, so the doping was clearly engineered to affect the outcome of the race, often without consideration for the health and safety of the animal. By contrast, the athlete usually (though not always) took their concoctions voluntarily. From the perspective of some trainers, the concoctions were specially designed supplements and their use provided a necessary stimulant to wake up or further motivate an already motivated athlete. Doping an animal was viewed as a different sort of deception. The English Jockey Club banned the doping of horses in 1903, and by 1910 they had developed saliva tests to detect the presence of banned drugs, including cocaine and heroin. By contrast, the International Amateur Athletic Federation (IAAF) did not formally ban doping among humans until 1928, and even then there were no tests of other enforcement procedures. Athletes just had to promise that they had not used any doping agents.

Amphetamines

The temptation to use artificial stimulants increased significantly after pharmaceutical companies began marketing them worldwide in the 1920s. The story began when Berlin University researcher Lazar Edeleano first synthesized phenylisopropylamine (later named **amphetamine**) in the late 1880s, though at the time he did not recognize its active properties. Almost concurrently, on the other side of the globe in Japan, a researcher working for Dainippon Pharmaceutical Company, Nagayoshi Nagai, discovered an adrenaline analogue that he identified as **ephedrine**. Within a few years, Nagai further synthesized a variant of ephedrine, which came to be known as **methamphetamine**. At that point, neither researcher recognized the stimulant effects of either variant.

After the First World War, both compounds were improved upon. In Japan, Nagai synthesized a crystal form of methamphetamine that made it easier to produce and to administer. Meanwhile, back in the United States, Gordan Alles was researching various insulin analogues as possible treatments for diabetes and stumbled across the physiological effects of both kinds of amphetamines. Alles sold his discovery to Smith, Kline & French, who marketed the drug as an inhaler (called Benzadrine) used to stimulate the respiratory system for the treatment of asthma. By the late 1920s, the inhalant form of amphetamine and the crystallized form of methamphetamines were recognized worldwide for their usefulness as a quick stimulant, outside their intended therapeutic purposes.

The nonspecific medical uses of amphetamines became popular during the 1930s, and physicians proscribed them for any number of mild to moderate treatments, including depression, weight gain, morning sickness, narcolepsy, and even as a treatment of post-intoxication hangovers. The relatively inexpensive drug did not appear to be addictive, and its casual use as a useful stimulant carried little scandal. Both the Allied and Axis governments distributed amphetamines to their soldiers to improve their alertness and concentration during conflict. Amphetamine use in amateur and professional sports was not widely discussed, but neither was it kept secret. During the 1950s, several Olympic athletes gave press interviews where they admitted freely that they used pep pills, which was an expected part of elite sports.

As long as stimulants were viewed by the public as a commonly used supplement which posed no harm to the athlete and did not predictably impact the outcome of the competition, then the drugs were largely ignored. Allegations of doping were still seen as a source of scandal, but both the athletes and the public generally associated such charges with harder drugs, like cocaine, heroin, or the extremely toxic strychnine. In 1950, after being accused of doping his athletes, a physician for the Danish Rowing Team defended himself by arguing that it "is not doping, it does not involve artificial stimulant, but is rather a supplement that restores natural requirements."

TESTOSTERONE AS A SCIENTIFIC EDGE IN COMPETITION

As the 1950s economic boom stimulated national and international interest in highly competitive sporting events, neither amphetamines nor anabolic steroids were necessarily viewed as unfair or unhealthy. The American Medical Association (AMA) warned about using testosterone as a medical therapy, and the drug gained a reputation as a less serious pharmaceutical alternative (seen as a catalyst of male vitality). But the public did not always share these views. More often anabolic steroids were set on a level marginally equivalent to powerful vitamins. At one point in his 1945 book *The Male Hormone*, Paul de Kruif speculated about how exciting it would be to see athletes using steroids. He explained, "We know how both the St. Louis Cardinals and the St. Louis Brownes have won championships supercharged by vitamins. It would be interesting to watch . . . a professional group that would try a systemic supercharge with testosterone."

Kruif presupposed the need for more specific clinical testing and physician oversight to protect the health of athletes, but he did not seem concerned about their potential for undermining the purity of competition.

Ziegler's Weightlifters

The use of testosterone as a performance enhancer emerged first during international competitions. By the early 1950s, informed trainers and coaches began to suspect that the Soviet weightlifting team was taking some kind of ergogenic drug because the Soviet team suddenly began to sweep medals in all categories. The American weightlifting coach, Bob Hoffman, vocalized his suspicions after the Soviets walked away with seven medals in the 1952 Olympics (including three gold and three silver), but he had no evidence to prove it. After a World Championship in 1954, Hoffman and the U.S. Team physician John Ziegler took one of the Soviet trainers out to a local tavern in Vienna and managed to get a vocal confirmation that the Soviet lifters were using testosterone—though the exact makeup of the compound was unknown.

Ziegler went back to the states and began working on his own testosterone analogue that could be sustained in the human system and, if possible, might be customized to retain fewer androgenic effects. Within a few years, Ziegler synthesized **methandrostenalone**, which is a precursor to testosterone. He sold the patent to Ciba Pharmaceuticals, which marketed the drug under the name of **Dianabol** in the form of little pink tablets. According to the label, the drug was intended to treat hypogonadic conditions where weight gain was needed, such as osteoporosis and dwarfism. From the start, however, Dianabol was always intended for competition.

Ziegler was a strong weightlifting enthusiast, but he was also a medical doctor and he initially approached the use of Dianabol as a clinical trial. He gave pills to three of his friends, Bill March, Jake Hitchens, and Tom Garcy, who trained with Ziegler at the York Barbell Club owned by Bob Hoffman. The test subjects were given 10 milligrams a day and were asked to keep detailed records of use and effects. He recommended variable doses according to the size of the athlete, and short-term cycles of six weeks on and five weeks off. In addition to the steroid, Ziegler also developed a specialized training device, which he combined with a high-protein diet to reach ideal effect. Taking anabolic steroids without training or the proteins produced few noticeable results. Yet, when combined with a high-intensity workout to stimulate muscle growth, the steroids used the high proteins to develop tissue growth. Over the course of several years, Ziegler's test subjects consistently won their international competitions.

Spread of Anabolic Steroids

As the news travelled, so too did Ziegler's methods. Very early on, Ziegler published an article in Hoffman's *Strength and Health* magazine describing a new training technique called "functional isometric contraction," to which he attributed the growing success of his lifters. Ziegler made no mention of Dianabol, but few were deceived and word spread about the drug's effectiveness nonetheless. As other trainers and competitors talked, Dianabol's popularity spread from coast to coast. By mid-decade, other pharmaceutical companies became involved and a host of testosterone variants were developed and sold by several competing companies. Their chemical names were fluoxymesterone, oxymetholone, oxymesterone, oxandrolone, norethandrolone, nandrolone phenpropionate, nandrolone decanoate, methandriol, bolasterone, ethylestrenol, and norbolethone. The product names were not necessarily any more accessible: Halotestin, Ultandren, Adroyd, Oranabol, Anavar, Nivelar, Durabolin, Deca-Durabolin, Stendiol, Myagen, Maxibolin, and Genabol. The male hormone was sold and used by millions legally and illegally worldwide.

Though anabolic steroids were initially intended for weightlifters, they were quickly adopted by other sports as well. About five years after Ziegler's discovery, one of his colleagues, Alvin Roy, was hired as the strength training coach for the San Diego Chargers. Roy was an advocate of Dianabol and he convinced the team coaches to provide free access to the players during training season at mealtimes. Players later recalled bowls of pink pills in the cafeteria and coaches reminding them to take their pills every day. The changes became noticeable very quickly, both physical and psychological. Players were stronger, but also more aggressive.

After about six weeks, some of the players became concerned by the changes, and after talking with their personal physicians, some players uncovered research warning that long-term use of steroids resulted in shrunken testicles, which indicated that the drugs were more powerful than they originally assumed. These players informed their coaches and after a team meeting, anabolic steroid use was cut back and access appeared to be more limited. Nevertheless, anabolic steroids were not abandoned altogether. Use throughout the National Football League (NFL) became more common as Alvin Roy moved from the Chargers to the Kansas City Chiefs, the Oakland Raiders, and the Dallas Cowboys. Similar anecdotes of coach-sponsored steroid use can be found for others sports, including baseball, cycling, and track and field.

Steroids and the Emerging Chemical Culture

Ziegler was initially very enthusiastic about the potential of anabolic steroids to improve athletic performance if administered under limited doses, but he was unprepared for the widespread mostly unsupervised use that came to dominate the sports community. He later explained that he did not realize (until it was too late) that "most lifters had such obsessive personalities." Ziegler's 5–10 milligram dosing schedule was largely ignored as lifters self-medicated with doses of 10 and 20 times the recommended schedule. Athletes in a variety of sports began to manifest a broad range of disorders, including impaired liver function. Within a decade of his initial discovery, Ziegler became a vocal opponent of anabolic steroids and categorically condemned them for athletes. But his comments came relatively late, and the demand was too strong. As the medical historian William Taylor vividly recounted, "On Southern California beaches bodybuilders wore T-shirts that read, *Dianabol, the Breakfast of Champions*."

In part, Ziegler's invention spread quickly because it entered the mainstream of high-level competitive sports right at the time that the chemical culture of the 1960s first began to emerge. Between the 1950s and the 1960s, synthetic drugs were not viewed with the same level of skepticism as they were even a decade later. Athletes, coaches, and the general public were more willing to accept drug use if it was presented as a pharmaceutical aid. Psychotropic drugs were prescribed and taken by a strong percentage of the population, and several hallucinogenic drugs were legal and were touted by some fringe groups for their psychological benefits. A new generation of youth was easily convinced that almost any health problem could be solved with a chemical solution. In this context, Ziegler developed and initially promoted analogue steroids as a useful new supplement. Its later popularity was almost inevitable considering the times.

In part, also, the spread of anabolic steroid use as a performance enhancer was reinforced as an unexpected side effect of the drug itself. Testosterone encourages more aggressive behaviors, and over the years, the testimonies from long-term users confirm that the aggressive tendencies also affect judgment and day to day decision making. Later research conducted by Charles Yesalis, Virginia Cowart, Bob Goldman, Patricia Bush, and others provide numerous accounts not only of quick tempers and explosive outbursts, but also of general distortion of priorities wherein the pursuit of winning overcomes all other concerns, including personal health and safety. When that priority shift occurs, then the natural inhibitions that encourage individual restraint are overcome. Perhaps Ziegler's observation that lifters had obsessive personalities reflected more the profile of the anabolic user than the particular characteristic of weightlifters. It was this risk of athlete's physical health combined with the noticeable changes in psychological motivation that most influenced public opinion (and the opinion of coaches, trainers, and athletes) to viewing steroids as not only unsafe, but also unfair. Steroid use was reduced to a simple question: should athletes who are unwilling to risk personal health be forced to compete against those who are?

Public Reaction

Pharmaceutical companies may have downplayed the harmful side effects of drugs like Benzadrine during the 1930s, but the excesses of the chemical culture of the 1960s provided ample evidence to the contrary. Amphetamines are highly addictive physically and psychologically. Food and Drug Administration (FDA) warnings include cardiovascular risks of increased heart rates and blood pressure that may lead to deterioration of the heart muscle, including possible risk of myocardial infraction (heart attack). Risks to the nervous system begin with strong headaches, dizziness, insomnia, and a variety of mood disorders, including euphoria as well as depression, anxiety, and general uneasiness, all of which could lead to involuntary motor and phonic movements (like Tourette's syndrome) or other psychotic episodes. Other risks include impotence, loss of libido, anorexia, weight loss, and other gastrointestinal symptoms. All these risks increase through extended use, and the addictive nature of amphetamines make abuse much more likely. Anabolic steroids carry with them an even longer list of risks, and as these and other drugs manifested themselves in international competitions, the public's concern over doping increased accordingly. When world-class athletes, in the prime of their conditions, succumbed on the field, then the dangers of ergogenic drugs became hard to ignore.

Deaths of Jensen and Simpson

The first death at an Olympics competition, of Francisco Lazaro in 1912, was heat related and not drug related. The second death, however, in 1960 was clearly drug induced. Danish cyclist Knud Jensen was racing in the 100 kilometer team trial during a 100-degree day in the Roman foothills when he became disoriented and crashed his bike. The 23-year-old Jensen never regained consciousness and died in the hospital less than a day later. The official cause was heat stroke, but the autopsy revealed traces of methamphetamines, nicotynal alcohol, and Ronicol, which is a drug intended to increase blood circulation. A trainer for the Danish Team later admitted that they routinely used Ronicol. Observers at the time debated whether or not the drugs or the conditions were ultimately responsible for Jensen's death. In hindsight, though, it was clear that the drugs removed the natural inhibitions (pain, fatigue, weakness) that would have prevented Jensen from pushing his body to such extreme limits. It was like removing the governor from an automobile's transmission, allowing the engine to exceed maximum revolutions per minute and burn up.

Jensen's death was only the most serious of a number of near-death incidents during a short span of years where athletes collapsed on the

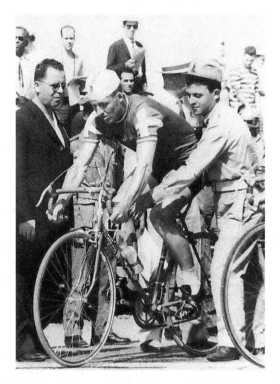

Danish cyclist Knud Enemark Jensen before the start of the 100-km team time trial at the Rome Olympics, August 26, 1960. During the race, Jensen collapsed with heat stroke and suffered a fractured skull, dying later in the hospital. His body tested positive for the drugs amphetamine and Roniacol at a subsequent autopsy. (Keystone/Hulton Archive/ Getty Images)

field, only to discover later that drugs were involved. An incident echoing Jensen occurred during the 1967 Tour de France, when English cyclist Tom Simpson died mid-race. He also began swerving and crashed at midday during a hill climb. Undaunted, he was helped back on the bike and continued on, only to collapse again just a short distance up the road. Later results indicated that he, too, used ergogenic drugs (amphetamines) to push his body beyond the natural inhibitions in an effort to win the race.

The physical health risks of drug use could be considered an individual decision if it were not for the psychological risks that seemed to accompany the abuse. When athletes push themselves so hard that they risk death to achieve victory, then that level of motivation affects the nature of the competition itself. What if an athlete, with perfectly natural priorities, preferred health and safety over winning, and therefore chose not to take the drugs? Does the nonusing athlete stand a fair chance in competition against drug-using athletes? As these questions became part of the public discussion during the mid-1960s, the governing authorities of national and international athletic associations began to address the problem of doping in sports more directly.

The Olympic Movement and Anti-Doping Rules

Within three months following Simpson's death, the IOC formed a Medical Commission to specifically address the problem of doping. Leaders on the Olympic movement had not been completely unaware of the problem. They were first alerted to the use of amphetamines in the 1930s, and after the Soviet weightlifting sweeps of the early 1950s, they became aware of anabolic steroids use. Yet, the threshold of urgency for IOC action did not become manifest until after Jensen's death—and even that tragedy succeeded only in launching planning initiatives. In 1966, advisors to the IOC recommended that a Medical Commission should be limited to providing expertise to local national affiliates so they could educate their athletes on the "moral and physical aspects of the drug problem." At that point, the IOC was advised to prepare facilities for the possibility of testing for drug use if the occasion arose, and to ensure proper sanctions if drug abuse became known. Otherwise, though, the IOC in 1966 was supposed to limit its action to simple condemnation. Simpson's death changed these plans significantly. The new Medical Commission of 1967 was expected to develop a specific list of banned substances, devise test procedures, and establish sanctions for violations.

GENDER AND COMPETITIVE EQUITY

The first meeting of the Medical Commission did not discuss doping but focused instead on procedures for instituting mandatory chromatin-based gender tests for the top three female winners in each of the women's events. The fear that men might compete disguised as women (or athletes suffering from **hermaphroditism**, which made the outward determination of gender less obvious) had been a concern of the IOC since 1936. Since the Olympic Games in Berlin, many observers became suspicious that some of the German female weightlifters were not actually women. Avery Brundage voiced those suspicions in 1936, and after he became IOC President in the 1960s, he made sure some measures were included in the new Medical Commission's rules. Nor were the fears unfounded. The two most suspicious athletes, Tamara and Irina Press (known as the Press Sisters) competed in track and field events for the Soviet Union and were both medalists in the 1960 and 1964 Olympic games. Both sisters withdrew from competition as soon as gender tests were implemented.

In modern games, this question remains significant. In countries that allow sex change operations, the use of anabolic steroid hormones is seen as a therapeutic treatment necessary for maintaining (or diminishing) male secondary sex traits. As a policy, the IOC will allow a therapeutic use exception in such cases, provided the treatments do not extend beyond the typical thresholds normally expected for men, and the athlete must compete as the new gender. The issue remains controversial and has not been tested through actual practice.

The deaths of Jensen and Simpson shifted public perception toward greater sensitivity to the dangers of ergogenic aids, and the mobilization of the IOC reflected the power of that new public pressure. In addition, though, the new concern for health safety also emphasized a parallel fear that athletes not wanting to endanger their lives for the sake of winning might face an unequal playing field when competing against athletes who do use drugs. The sense of fairness or the desire to ensure an equal playing field is what motivated the rules for both doping and gender tests. Women should not have to compete against men who are biologically stronger by nature due to their dominant testosterone ratio. Nor should women be pressured to take drugs that would alter their hormone ratios just so they could compete with equal chance as those who naturally produce those testosterone levels. The 1967 Medical Commission explicitly linked gender tests with doping tests because they viewed both as safeguards against unequal competition. The list of banned substances for the 1968 Olympic Games included:

1. Sympathomimetic amines (amphetamines)
2. Stimulants to the central nervous system (strychnine)
3. Narcotics and analgesics (morphine)
4. Antidepressants (imipramine)
5. Tranquilizers (phenothiazine)

Anabolic steroids were not included in the list. They were recognized as a major problem, but in 1967, there were no tests available to check for them. It was not until 1973 that the technology of ergogenic detection momentarily caught up the technology of rational design. Using an extremely expensive gas liquid chromatography mass spectronomy machine, the IOC could detect anabolic steroids in athletes (or at least one of the 17 steroid variants currently available at that time). Only at that point were anabolic steroids formally added to the list of banned substances (though, perhaps ironically, not testosterone—because it was still undetectable). As the Medical Commission explained in 1974, "The reason for banning [anabolic steroids] is not only because their use contravenes sporting ethics but because it constitutes a definite danger to females and also to the growth of young people." The commission went on to list other specific risks, including liver damage, sterility in men, and greater chances of cancer.

By the 1970s, the public perception of anabolic steroids (and all ergogenic drugs) changed significantly enough to take for granted that their use constituted a breach of competitive fairness and equal opportunity. The health risks of stimulant abuse had become obvious by the 1960s, but it was not until the 1970s that the same recognition was extended to anabolic steroids. Once the health risk was clearly embraced by the general public and the expectation of fair competition reaffirmed, then amateur sports reacted accordingly. In 1972, the IOC Charter was amended to include an explicit condemnation of "the use of drugs or artificial stimulants of any kind." Two years later, the Charter was amended again to explicitly warn athletes that such drug use (or even refusal to take drug tests) would result in elimination. The Olympic movement was taking specific steps to ensure that Pierre de Coubertin's dream of pure, amateur sport remained untainted from the corruption that surrounded the professionals of his day. Yet, the professional sports organizations in the 1980s and 1990s were having a much more difficult time of ensuring such similar safeguards.

THE RACE BETWEEN EVASION AND DETECTION: TESTOSTERONE, BLOOD DOPING, hGH, AND DESIGNER STEROIDS

Just six years after the IOC adopted its more aggressive anti-doping policies, the 1980 Olympic Games earned the unique distinction of having zero athletes test positive for banned substances. Neither the winter games in Lake Placid nor the summer games in Moscow were tarnished by the scandal of ergogenic drug use. That, of course, does not mean that all athletes were drug free. Anecdotal evidence from observers at that time and from testimonies after the fact indicated that a great number of athletes were using some form of performance-enhancing drug. There is a general consensus that the amount of drug use likely increased from 1976 to 1980. What was unique, though, was that not a single athlete was caught.

The lag between when a new ergogenic drug is introduced and when a cost-effective detection method is developed always provides athletes with an advantage. In the 1970s, the IOC anti-doping labs were able to detect synthetic androgenic anabolic steroids by measuring the presence of certain substituent chains that are not native to human systems. There were no specific tests for testosterone itself, because testosterone naturally occurs in the body and scientists had not (yet) developed tests to distinguish between testosterone that was synthesized naturally by the body and the testosterone that was administered externally. One of the unintended consequences of IOC tests for synthetic anabolic steroids was that it prompted some athletes to apply testosterone directly to targeted muscle groups. By that time, delivery methods for testosterone included gels and films that were applied topically as an ointment (or as a patch) directly above the target muscles and suspensions that were injected directly into the targeted muscle. As long as the athlete stopped the doping prior to competition, the IOC testing methods of 1980 were not able to detect the testosterone.

Testosterone Testing

Officials involved with the international anti-doping community were not deceived by the lack of positive results during the 1980 Olympics. Players had been caught with anabolic steroids in the years leading up to the games and they continued to be caught in different international venues after the games. Recognizing that a loophole must exist somewhere, the IOC employed a new method developed by Manfred Donike that measured the ratio of glucuroconjugated testosterone to epitestosterone (also known as **T/E ratio**) in urine. Epitestosterone is a hormone that has almost the exact structure of testosterone, except that the—OH group on the C17 position points in the opposite direction. Under natural conditions, the two hormones are produced by the testes simultaneously, so most people will have a 1:1 ratio at any given time. The epitestosterone levels do not change when testosterone is introduced from outside the body, so if an athlete demonstrated a T/E ratio of 6:1 or higher, then the IOC assumed that it was caused by artificial means. The T/E ratio is not absolute, insofar as it does not identify the specific drug used to elevate the testosterone levels. Nevertheless, for the purposes of international anti-doping officials, it was sufficient to demonstrate that doping had occurred.

The first use of the T/E ratio test occurred at the Pan American Games held in Caracas, Venezuela, in 1983. Coaches were warned that a new test was being developed that was significantly more sensitive and that athletes would be tested immediately after each competition. That year, an unusually high number of athletes chose to stay home at the last moment. The news became a scandal after the first day of the games, when word spread among the contestants that several athletes tested positive for steroid use. Almost immediately, there was a rash of illnesses and dozens of athletes suddenly chose to go home (rather than face the inevitable testing). In the end, 19 athletes from 10 countries were disqualified, resulting in 23 medals passed along to the next competing athletes. More than a dozen Americans left the games voluntarily. The scandal captured headlines throughout the world and athletes were put on notice that doping for international competitions would be much more difficult to hide.

Individual Evasion

Individual athletes, especially, found the new testing procedures used at international competitions to be difficult to evade—though not impossible. If individual athletes limited their steroid use during training seasons only and ended their treatment cycles early enough prior to the next competition (or next drug testing), then they stood a good chance of evading detection. This method was not precise because the individual athlete had no way of knowing with certainty how sensitive the new testing tools were or how many traces of their ergogenic drug might still be left in their system. As a result, individual athletes working in isolation frequently got caught. Later, after the World Anti-Doping Agency (WADA) took over testing procedures, athletes were subject to random testing any time of the year. These new precautions made evasion among isolated athletes much more difficult.

The situation, however, was different when athletes, coaches, and medical experts worked in collusion to evade detection. Almost immediately following the Pan American Games in 1983, East German scientists began developing techniques and methods for more reliable evasion. Since the

1950s, the small communist country used international sports competition as a medium for Cold War propaganda, and they placed a great deal of emphasis on winning a disproportionate number of medals given their population size. Years later, after the fall of the Soviet Union, documents emerged which revealed that the East German sports director, Dr. Manfred Höeppner, authorized the use of anabolic steroids for all sports fields as early as 1970. The coaches successfully avoided detection by carefully managing a regimen of internal testing and experimentation.

The athletes were told to cooperate or face expulsion from the program. It is likely that many of the East German athletes did not know what they were taking, and if they suspected it, they did not say anything for fear of retribution from their own government. The East German labs in Kreischa earned approval as an IOC testing site, and local officials gained inside information on procedures and thresholds. The team doctors tested athletes routinely to find out precisely when evidence of steroids left their system. If traces remained at the time of completion, the athlete would become ill and stay home. The IOC relied on local national committees to report results of their testing. If a local committee was corrupt, then there was little the international community could do to uncover the abuse.

Blood Doping

The organized subversion of anti-doping procedures produced a number of other ergogenic alternatives that were not initially available to individual athletes. In the early 1970s, a Swedish doctor, Bjorn Ekblöm, discovered that athletes could improve their endurance up to 25 percent if they packed their blood with higher-than-normal red blood cell ratios. The procedure, called **blood doping**, rests on the fact that red blood cells carry oxygen to muscles, which impacts both endurance and performance.

Individuals cannot engage in blood doping without help. The procedure requires technical training as doctors draw oxygenated blood and then reinject it into the athlete prior to competition. Transfusions between different people (called **homologous blood doping**) may lead to serious, sometimes lethal, consequences if the blood is not carefully tested and screened for compatibility and other pathogens. Athletes may use their own oxygenated blood (called **autologous blood** doping), but they must be able to store it safely and they still require sanitary procedures for reinjection. Both methods require willing collaboration between the athlete, their trainer, and a qualified medical professional.

Blood doping was legal in the 1970s, but remained secret because most competitors recognized that it violated the spirit of anti-doping ideal, and the public would not likely be supportive. The IOC eventually banned blood-doping in 1986, but scientists were still unable to effectively test for it. Though methods existed to detect homologous blood doping, there were no methods for detecting autologous blood doping because it does not involve any nonnative molecules. Blood doping improves endurance, but it does not have significant impact on more immediate performance needs. As such, the ergogenic tool has been most associated with long distance cyclists, runners and swimmers. In 2012, scientists were able to detect RNA differences between fresh blood and stored blood, and the following year Lance Armstrong—winner of an unprecedented seven consecutive Tour de France races between 1999 and 2006—was caught using blood doping (among other ergogenic tools).

EPO and hGH

By the end of the 1980s, some of the methods that had been developed through team collusion began to spill out among individual athletes again. A Massachusetts company, Amgen, refined a glycoprotein hormone called recombinant erythropoietin, which had been isolated and discovered nearly 20 years earlier. Amgen marketed the drug under the name of Epogen (also called **EPO**), which was approved by the FDA as a treatment for anemia. Almost immediately, athletes within the sports community adapted the drug as a synthetic form of blood doping. The hormone increased the number of red blood cells and achieved the same results. It was not detectable until the early 2000s, and the drug became especially popular among cyclists. Unfortunately, oxygen-rich blood is also thicker and often leads to heart attacks, blood clots, and strokes. Between 1987 and 1989, 15 professional cyclists died under unexplained circumstances, which many observers attributed to EPO.

In addition to EPO, athletes also gained access to synthetic Human Growth Hormones (also called **hGH**) in the mid-1980s. The polypeptide hormone is synthesized by the pituitary gland, and is responsible for new cell production and bone growth. The hormone converts insulin into a growth factor for bones, muscles, and other tissues. It was isolated and characterized as early as the 1930s, but unlike other hormones, hGH seemed to be species specific. That meant that it could not be harvested from another plant or nonmammalian animal. The hormone had to be harvested directly from the pituitary glands of cadavers, which significantly limited both supply and research potential into therapeutic applications. From the 1950s, hGH was used as a treatment for children afflicted with dwarfism, until doctors in the 1980s discovered a link between natural hGH and a fatal neurological disorder known as **Creutzfeldt-Jakob disease**. American pharmaceutical company, Genentech, responded by developing a synthetic form of hGH in 1985 to eliminate the Creutzfeldt-Jakob risk, and marketed the drug under the name of Nutropin. The supply of synthetic hGH increased significantly, which proved a benefit to children suffering from slow physical growth. At the same time, athletes also quickly recognized its potential as a substitute for testosterone-based anabolic steroids, seemingly without the androgenic side effects.

The FDA approved the synthetic hGH (Nutropin) as a therapeutic treatment for very serious conditions in both children and adults. In addition to impeded bone growth, hGH also treats Turners Syndrome in girls, **Prader-Willi Syndrome**, and other symptoms related to kidney insufficiency. For adults, hGH can be used to treat deficiencies caused by pituitary tumors and AIDS/HIV patients suffering from muscle-wasting disease. The treatment is not without side effects, including edema (swelling), carpal tunnel syndrome, and other joint, nerve, and muscle pains, and numbness. The more severe side effects include increased cholesterol levels, increased risks of diabetes, **acromegaly** (enlarged bone growth, "gigantism"), and cancerous tumors. These risks increase significantly in patients without preexisting pituitary deficiencies.

Nutropin manufacturer, Genentech, kept tight controls over its supplies; nevertheless, the drug still found its way into the athletic community as a black market performance enhancer. Initially, the illicit supply had to be the result of complicit doctors, who illegally prescribed the drug for non-listed purposes, or simply created fake patients to enable distributors to sell to dealers around the country. Only a few corrupt doctors would be needed to supply thousands of athletes with hGH, thereby undermining rigid restrictions imposed by the manufacturers. The temptation was high, because the black market was a very lucrative business, with some athletes reportedly paying $500 a week for their hGH supply. Very quickly, the demand for the drug far exceeded the natural demand created from children and adults suffering from targeted symptoms. Other drug manufacturers responded by entering the market, including Eli Lilly (marketing Humatrope in 1987), Novo Nordisk (marketing Norditropin in 1988), Teva (marketing Tev-Tropin in 1995), Pfizer (marketing Genotropin in 1995), and Serono (marketing Saizen in 2000). By the turn of the millennium, hGH was widely available, though still highly regulated.

Designer Steroids

Reports of hGH use among professional athletes increased significantly in the 1990s. Aside from the potential of achieving tissue growth similar to anabolic steroids without the resulting secondary sex characteristics, the other perceived benefit was that hGH was undetectable by anti-doping testing procedures within the international sports community. It was a poorly kept secret since most officials knew of its widespread use. In the late 1980s alone, there were several books published detailing the various forms of ergogenic drugs and techniques, including EPO, hGH, and other anabolic steroids. Yet, without reliable detection methods, there was little that anti-doping officials could do to stop the tide of use. The IOC did not unveil a blood test for hGH until the 2004 games in Athens, but even then the test could not reliably detect the drug if it was taken more than 48 hours prior. A urine-based test was developed in 2008, which could detect hGH used within two weeks, but no labs were set up to effectively test players on a routine basis. More reliable and cost-effective tests for hGH were only discovered in the 2010s. Their implementation in 2012–2013 created significant controversy among sports associations (Major League Baseball [MLB], National Basketball Association [NBA], and NFL), presumably because of the suspected widespread use of hGH among professional athletes.

In the meantime, during the mid-1980s, Victor Conte opened up a business in the San Francisco Bay Area that specialized in assessing the condition of athletes, and prescribing a customized list of supplements to address weak points and improve overall fitness. The company, called the Bay Area Laboratory Co-Operative (**BALCO**), initially focused on herbal and other dietary supplements. As the available biotechnology became more sophisticated, BALCO expanded into biochemical engineering. For a price, even isolated athletes could go to a business that would help them improve their performance, without necessarily involving game officials or even team coaches/managers. In 1999, BALCO developed the first **designer steroid**, norbolethone, which was deliberately designed to avoid detection by existing anti-doping procedures. Norbolethone was not identified by anti-doping officials until 2002. From the perspective of officials in the global anti-doping community, this discovery gave proof that conspiracies to evade detection could occur even at the individual level.

THE WILL TO POLICE: WADA REGULATIONS AND LEGAL PROHIBITIONS

In terms of technological development, the anti-doping detectives will always lag behind the users seeking evasion. Yet, the success of an individual athlete is largely based on their ability to find willing accomplices to help them. As long as the international sports community desired drug-free competition, then the only way they could limit the extent of evasion was to limit the opportunity for large-scale conspiracies to subvert the anti-doping system. To be successful, the will to enforce anti-doping regulations needed to extend beyond the minority of international officials and be embraced at all levels, including national and local cooperation. That would require a culture of anti-doping. International officials establish procedures to oversee national authorities, but only the civil authorities of each nation can implement laws that would regulate private enterprises (like BALCO) from engaging in the same sorts of doping conspiracy.

Festina Scandal

Among amateur associations, the IOC led the way in establishing global standards for anti-doping regulations. Yet, even their leadership was prompted by a constant stream of public scandals among international competitors. The 1990s were filled with news stories of elite athletes (runners, cyclists, swimmers, etc.) failing to pass drug tests—the *New York Times* featured more than 500 such stories during that time period. Individual scandal was disheartening, but the prospect of national level conspiracy seemed to most seriously challenge the integrity of international competition. The East German machine during the 1980s and the Chinese swimmer scandal of 1994 were not entirely unexpected, since both countries were ruled by totalitarian regimes that routinely issued public statements that seemed to manipulate the truth—deception in national sports was not incongruous with other examples of national propaganda. Yet, when similar levels of conspiracy spread into the west, the public reaction was much stronger.

The **Festina Scandal** during the 1998 Tour de France seemed to confirm the existence of coordinated evasion among teams from Western Democracies. During a routine border patrol check, a car operated by the French Cycling Team on its way to the Tour de France competition was caught carrying a large supply of ergogenic drugs, including EPO, hGH, steroids, and other masking agents designed to evade detection. The seizure captured national attention in France, and the local police launched a series of searches among other national cycling teams, which eventually implicated the Dutch, Spanish, and Italian teams. Images of police carrying suitcases filled with seized drugs and escorting coaches and players away in cuffs plagued the reputation of the race. In the end, barely half the riders remained to finish the Tour de France due to doping-related complications. The prospect that so many national level officials participated in more or less open conspiracies to evade detection of ergogenic drugs suggested an unwillingness of the governing organization to police its own competitions.

World Anti-Doping Agency

The Tour de France officials were highly embarrassed and they vowed to be much more proactive in the future, and they pledged a zero-tolerance policy in subsequence races. Public pressure for action did not end in France, though, and the IOC responded to the Festina Scandal by introducing a new system of enforcement that did not rely as heavily on national cooperation. Just months before the turn of the new millennium, the IOC launched the WADA as an independent entity charged with setting the standards for drug-free competition among all international athletes, and for the testing and enforcement of those standards. Almost all international level sports associations follow guidelines established by WADA and use WADA-approved drug-testing labs. As the new WADA Code explained, its purpose was to "protect the athlete's fundamental right to participate in doping-free sport and thus promote health, fairness, and equality for athletes worldwide." In this way, the independent agency would serve as a watchdog of both individual athletes and national organizations.

The WADA created the public pressure necessary to encourage individual nations to cooperate. Organized attempts to evade detection continued to be unmasked within international competition, but voluntary participation in WADA provided individual national sports programs with the opportunity to prove that they were not responsible for the malfeasance, and their policies reflected their commitment to drug-free competition. The reputation and integrity of each nation's sports authorities required evidence of comprehensive safeguards that made evasion more difficult. Throughout the 1980s and 1990s, countries dealt with the problem of steroid abuse in different ways, but ultimately almost every government around the globe publicly prohibited the sale of anabolic steroids for nontherapeutic usage.

Each nation's prohibition against anabolic steroids demonstrated to the rest of the world their commitment to drug-free competition at all levels—not just at the international venues. Nevertheless, some significant disparity exists between nations. France became the first country to list certain ergogenic drugs as illegal in 1963 (in response to the back-to-back Jensen and Smith tragedies). The United Kingdom is unique among western nations by prohibiting the purchase and supply of anabolic steroids, but not forbidding possession for personal use. Mexico permits the sale of steroids with a prescription, but local pharmacies rarely request evidence of them. Indeed, many non-Western countries prohibit anabolic steroids and yet ignore prevailing black market trades. Thailand, for example, is often incorrectly thought to have legalized anabolic steroids, but on paper the Thai

Food and Drug law prohibiting possession and sale of steroids carries a stiff jail sentence. In actual practice, though, steroids are easily obtained there. Mexico, China, and Thailand are often cited as major production sources of supply for the illegal ergogenic drug trade.

American Sports Entertainment

In the United States, the legal status of anabolic steroids evolved throughout the 1980s as public attention over expulsion of elite athletes during international meets became increasingly common. Technically, Congress prohibited the prescription of anabolic steroids for nontherapeutic purposes in the Food, Drug and Cosmetic Act of 1980, but at that time violation carried no criminal penalty. It was not until the passage of the Anti-Drug Abuse Act of 1988 that criminal penalties were applied.

One of the difficulties of explicit prohibition in the United States was that the market for sports-related competition often conflicted with sports-related entertainment. For example, Professional Wrestling emerged with the advent of television as a popular American entertainment alternative in the 1950s. Each network included professional wrestling programs in their weekly lineup, and the genre eliminated actual competition in favor of colorful storylines and scripted performances. After a hiatus during the 1970s, professional wrestling reemerged in the 1980s by such promoters as Vince McMahon and by star performers such as Hulk Hogan. McMahon openly described the programming of his World Wrestling Federation (WWF) as sports entertainment. The popularity was due not only to the live action of the performances, but also to the competitor's large muscular physiques. Hogan later admitted to receiving regular supplies of anabolic steroids from McMahon throughout his career. Hogan believed they were legal because they were prescribed by a doctor. Both McMahan and Hogan believed that anti-doping policies were inappropriate for Professional Wrestlers because there was very little competition in the sport, the primary purpose for the anabolic steroids was cosmetic—not competitive performance enhancement.

Similar trends of action-based entertainment dominated other cultural centers in the United States. After winning the Mr. Universe title at the age of 20 and later the Mr. Olympia bodybuilding contest (seven times), Arnold Schwarzenegger became a major box office draw in films such as *Conan the Barbarian*, *The Terminator*, and more than 40 other movies. Schwarzenegger was known for his huge muscles, which he openly attributed to a routine, though moderate, use of anabolic steroids. Other action-based actors like Sylvester Stallone (of *Rocky*, *Rambo*, and more than 60 other movies) also used testosterone to build up giant muscles for their character's performances. Hollywood's demand for talented strong-men created significant incentive for steroid use among performers. When used for purely entertainment purposes, the American public seemed to have little concern about anabolic steroid use. Yet, at the same time, the public became increasingly less tolerant of ergogenic drugs when used for purposes of gaining a competitive advantage. During much of the 1980s, the conflicting messages left American lawmakers somewhat ambivalent on reinforcing existing prohibitions.

Entertainment and Professional Sports Associations

One of the triggers for change occurred toward the end of the decade. During the 1988 Summer Olympics in Seoul, Korea, Canadian sprinter Ben Johnson was stripped of his world record and gold medal for his 100 meter sprint after failing his drug test. Traces of stanozolol were found in his system, and Johnson's gold medal, title, and new Olympic record was passed along to the American runner Carl Lewis. The news dominated American headlines, and a month later President Reagan signed the Anti-Drug Abuse Act of 1988. The law focused primarily on drug smuggling, gang violence, rehabilitation, and other measures involved in narcotics trafficking; yet, a small provision was included that added criminal penalties for prescribing anabolic steroids without a prescription. Two years later, the elder Bush administration signed the Anabolic Steroids Control Act of 1990, which reclassified the drug as a Schedule III controlled substance. That category includes drugs that are currently used by the medical community to address legitimate therapeutic purposes, but for which there is also a high risk of abuse leading either to low physical dependence or to high psychological dependence. Other drugs in this category include meth-amphetamines, amphetamines, opium, and morphine. The federal government outlawed steroids, but enforcing the law remained another issue.

From the perspective of the American legal system, anabolic steroids were publicly prohibited and controlled by 1990. Nevertheless, evidence suggested that society's will to actively enforce these laws remained weak throughout the 1990s. While the anti-doping testing procedures for international competitions became increasingly sophisticated (eventually resulting in the creation of WADA), the professional sports associations in the United States seemed much more resistant to change. The NFL was the first association to ban steroids in 1983, and it was the first to suspend players in 1989 after it began testing for illegal substances. Suspensions, however, ranged from four games for first offence up to a year for third offense. This is significantly less than the guidelines set by WADA, which includes a two-year suspension for first offence and lifetime ban for second.

The NBA did not formally ban steroid use until 1999, and then testing remains limited to four random tests throughout the year, with penalties ranging from 5-game suspension for first offense to a maximum penalty of 25-game suspension for fourth offence (or more). Though MLB tacitly reminded club owners that all illegal substances were banned (and steroids for nontherapeutic use were illegal in 1990), the association did not begin testing for drug use until 2003, with penalties ranging from a 10-day suspension for first offense to a 1-year suspension for fourth offence.

Observers continue to debate whether professional sports associations in the United States are genuinely committed to policing anti-doping policies that are officially on the books. The entertainment value of hard-pounding linemen, record-breaking home run hitters, and sky-high slam dunks is difficult to distinguish from the sense of fairness associated with drug-free competition. Professional sports teams are businesses as much as they are venues of competition, and the public demand for exciting performances often challenges the sportsmen's desire for fair and equitable play. One of the factors that helped to change the trend was the fear of public disapproval. The NFL rational for its anti-doping policies lists not only a desire to maintain the integrity of playing field first, but it also includes concerns about protecting the player's health and ensuring that the "wrong message" is not sent "to young people who may be tempted to use" anabolic steroids modeling after their sports heroes. Perhaps, the most significant incentives for professional accommodation to anti-doping policy came from public pressure to ensure a family friendly entertainment.

In 2000, shortly after the formation of WADA, the American authorities organized the United States Anti-Doping Agency (**USADA**) to serve as an independent body to ensure the integrity and commitment of amateur sports associations. Professional sports association did not necessarily follow USADA guidelines. Nevertheless, news of BALCO's designer drugs, coupled with a series of scandals among leading baseball players during the early 2000s, pressured all professional sports associations in the United States to increase the sophistication of their anti-doping policies. Regardless of the personal preferences of owners, managers, and coaches within individual sports associations, the rigor of existing testing procedures became increasingly difficult to evade.

CONCLUSION

Legends are filled with stories of secret brews, or spells, or other fountains of youth that promise to evade the pains of old age. In the modern age, brews and spells have been replaced by science and technology, and the fabled dream is still just as compelling as it was in ancient times. If there was a drug that guaranteed even 100 years of extra life, then there would be few people who would resist the temptation to take it, even if the drug was expensive and even if the drug was illegal. For almost a century, scientists have turned to biochemistry and the field of anabolic steroids in the hope of discovering a physiological solution to the time-honored pursuit of evading old age.

Health Concerns

The problem is that anabolic steroids do not affect the whole person and they cannot control the system-wide cycle that determines growth and decay. Testosterone and other related anabolic steroid hormones can maintain the kind of muscle growth that is most associated with youth, but they do not have similar impact on the other systems. Bones and joints, the brain and its nervous system, the heart and its circulatory system, digestion, and a host of other interrelated components working together are all responsible for the natural cycle of youth and eventual old age and decline. Users may seek youth during their declining years or may seek to multiply their growth potential during their youthful years, but in each case the use of anabolic steroids is limited by a plethora of other interrelated interactions that scientists, as yet, do not fully understand. What happens when the skeletal system of a 44-year-old is faced with a muscular system of a 20-year-old? How does that impact joints, ligaments, and other areas? Similarly, what happens when a 20-year-old doubles or triples the amount of muscular pressure that their body normally accommodates—how does the multiplied workload impact the cardiovascular system or the increase in metabolic activity impact digestive system? There is little question that anabolic steroids and other ergogenic drugs improve performance in both strength and endurance, but that improvement always comes at a cost to other areas of the body. As of yet, anabolic steroids can only affect one small part of the complex physiological network and there is no magical fountain of youth that evades the onset of age-related pathologies.

The main controversy related to anabolic steroid use for performance enhancement always boils down to questions of health and safety. If the use of tissue-building hormones were always safe, then they would be classified in the same categories as vitamins and healthy dietary supplements. Indeed, when they were first introduced to the weight-lifting community during the early years of the chemical revolution, anabolic steroids and other ergogenic aids carried little social stigma, and the athletic community was hesitant to question their value for training and conditioning. Public opinion changed once athletes in the prime of their condition began to succumb in the field of competition or were found dead with unusual high amounts of ergogenic chemicals in their systems. Questions of competitive fairness followed after questions of medical safety had already begun to surface. Was it fair for an athlete, with natural concerns about long-term health, to face a competitive disadvantage because others do not share that same concern? The question of competitive equality rests on the presumption that all athletes have a right to compete without being forced to risk their personal well-being in order to have a chance at winning.

Similarly, health and safety also underlie the pressure behind legal prohibitions against noncompetitive use of anabolic steroids for cosmetic purposes. Professional wrestlers and Hollywood action heroes may not face the pressure of unscripted competition, but they serve as role models for millions of young people who do. The giant physical size of these media icons are impossible without some kind of ergogenic supplement, and there is a strong possibility that a teen may underestimate the dangers and health risks associated with those performance-enhancing drugs because their heroes appear to use them without ill effect. Other, more competitive, professional sports associations also recognized the risks to youth of poor modeling, and took steps to publicly denounce anabolic steroids—even when the consequences threatened to impact their economic bottom line. The national consensus of health risks associated with such drugs, created public pressure for anti-doping precautions in noncompetitive venues. Lawmakers responded accordingly, and they criminalized the nontherapeutic use of anabolic steroids. The public record reflects disapproval of any socioeconomic pressure that might induce someone to place their personal health and well-being in jeopardy for the sake of temporary physical advantage.

Therapeutic Stigma

The public association of anabolic steroids with performance enhancement is so strong that it has impacted other research into therapeutic applications. William Taylor first gained national prominence during the 1980s with a series of books exposing the harmful health effects of anabolic steroids among competitive athletes. His books, *Anabolic Steroids and the Athlete* (1982), *Hormonal Manipulation: A New Era of Monstrous Athletes* (1985), and *Macho Medicine: A History of the Anabolic Steroid Epidemic* (1992) earned him a prominent place in national discussion of more effective anti-doping policies and legal prohibitions. Taylor is included among a list of doctors and research academics who are labeled "crusaders" in the fight for more rigid procedures in the testing and monitoring of steroid abuse in amateur and professional sports. Other names included in this list as Gary Wadler, Charles Yesalis, Richard Melloni, and Robert Cantu.

Despite his impressive credentials as an opponent of ergogenic drug use in sports competition, Taylor also argues that anabolic steroids has earned an unfair reputation. His 2002 book, *Anabolic Therapy in Modern Medicine*, identified 30 areas where anabolic steroids could provide potential advantage as a therapeutic treatment. Some of the disorders he discussed include an array of autoimmune diseases, sarcopenia, and osteoporosis, and some potential rehabilitation therapies include hormone replacement and supplemental support for common catabolic steroid treatment options. Taylor's point was that the public scandals among competitive athletes caused researchers to be more hesitant to investigate traditional therapeutic applications of the androgenic effects of anabolic steroids for fear that the research would by dismissed (or abused) by patients and doctors.

Renewed Search for Fountain of Youth

Serious researchers often hesitate to become associated with the pseudoscience of antiaging remedies. Like Charles Brown-Ségard claiming to have discovered the elixir for eternal youth, the public is both wary and tempted by unrealistic marketing claims promising to extend male vitality. Despite the possible taint of medical entrepreneurialism, the market for antiaging supplements is often too strong to resist. Consumers spent more than $44 billion on cosmetic body care and facial care products in 2012, and two-thirds of that money was spent by people aged 25 and over. The specific market for curative antiaging products for people aged 45 and over was $4.2 billion and just slightly less at $3.1 billion for people aged 35–44. These cosmetic products do not include the less-regulated market for herbal supplements and the uncounted black market for inappropriately used ergogenic drugs for cosmetic purposes. In part, the increase in demand is due to an aging baby boomer population, which anticipates 10,000 people turning 50 years every day from 2010 to 2025. The fear of growing (or looking) old accounts, in part, for the 10 million new gym membership every year (45 million in total, resulting in 4.6 billion visits a year). The health club market grew from $19.5 billion in 1994 to $67.2 billion in 2009. Similarly, the growing internet has responded to aging baby boomers with increasing proportion of retailers advertising testosterone, hGH, and other ergogenic drugs as antiaging remedies that "make you look and feel younger." The market for herbal supplements that invigorate increased from $4 billion in 1994 to $23.7 billion in 2008, with more than 5 percent of sales occurring online. Not surprising, two of the most advertised drugs in 2012, Cialis (by Eli Lilly, $162 million) and Viagra (by Pfizer, $107 million) both treat erectile dysfunction, which is most associated with old age.

Despite the increasingly proactive anti-doping policies among sports associations, the demand among the general public for a secret (perhaps an unregulated or illegal) formula to extend youthful performance has not diminished. In 2002, the Florida FDA office issued warnings to web-based retailers who claimed that people who use hGH (marketed as Saizen) see "15% average decrease in fat . . . 8% average increase in muscle and lean body structure." Other claims included improved libido, better sleep patterns, stronger bones, fewer wrinkles, and improved cardiac and kidney functions—essentially all the characteristics of youth. The FDA reiterated the fact that hGH is only approved for "the long-term treatment of children with growth failure due to inadequate secretion of endogenous growth hormone." The FDA also warned that continued advertising of such claims would result in criminal penalties, seizure, injunctions, and imprisonment of up to five years in a federal prison. Nevertheless, prosecution is extremely difficult. This example is one of thousands of other similar websites, adverting both prescription and over-the-counter drugs to restore youthful vitality. The FDA does not have the resources to police the wide multitude of media formats.

The black market sales notwithstanding, the legal market for anabolic steroids also increased in the 2010s. The sales of legally prescribed testosterone replacement drugs such as Axiron (from Eli Lilly) and Androgel (from Abbot Labs) reached $2 billion in 2012, with a projected growth of $5 billion by 2017. Testosterone as a performance-enhancing drug is listed as a Schedule III controlled substance, but when prescribed by a doctor to treat a specific deficiency, the drug becomes a legal therapy. If a man is diagnosed with low testosterone, their levels fall below anticipated ranges and a doctor can legally prescribe testosterone without fear of violating the ban on ergogenic usage. The question remains, however, whether low testosterone exists as a genuine ailment or whether it is manufactured by pharmaceutical companies as an antiaging treatment. The body's natural production of testosterone decreases over time, resulting in such symptoms as loss of libido, decreased muscle/bone mass, and depression. Most of these symptoms are also reflective of old age, and some critics argue the low testosterone diagnosis is another term for old age. As the baby boomer generation reaches old age, the use of anabolic steroids as a tool of lifestyle enhancement may overcome their more common use as a performance enhancer for competition.

In part, the larger issue related to noncompetitive use of anabolic steroids is most related to other cultural trends that promote ideals of physical perfection. For example, public acceptance of elective cosmetic surgery has changed significantly between the 1960s and 2010s. Numerous polls in the 2010s indicated that more than half of the Americans would undergo plastic surgery if money was not an option, and among women the statistic often spiked as high as 70 percent. In 2012, the annual poll conducted by the American Academy of Facial Plastic and Reconstructive Surgeons among its 752 members indicated facial plastic surgeries for all reasons increased significantly from 2011 to 2012, and almost three quarters of these procedures (73%) were conducted for cosmetic and not reconstructive purposes). Perhaps, most surprising was the 28 percent increase in procedures conducted on women aged 13–19 years (a jump from 132,000 in 2011 to 169,000 in 2012). This statistic may also correspond with a 31 percent increase in the number of patients who wanted plastic surgery after viewing unfavorable pictures posted through social media photo sharing sites on the internet.

Some critics contend that the increasing exposure of social media in our contemporary media-oriented culture places excessive attention on physical beauty, which encourages people to pursue impossible ideals of perfection at all costs. Young girls are faced with thousands of pictures of cosmetically altered photographs, suggesting that beauty is determined by perfect shapes or other exterior characteristics. Nevertheless, other polls of popular opinion indicate that more than 60 percent of women believe plastic surgery is a right that any individual should have access to in order to combat their personal insecurities. One poll conducted by the readers of *More!* magazine (which targets women aged 40 and over), indicated that 35 percent of their readers believed plastic surgery should be free and included under any national health care plan. Critics of the youth-oriented mass media culture do not appear to be dominating the public debate. The association of anabolic steroids as a potential fountain of youth fits easily into either side of that discussion.

Moral Questions

In part, the public controversy associated with anabolic steroids reflects larger philosophical questions about cultural priorities and the balance between material health, physical appearance, and moral propriety. Not everyone supports anti-doping rules for competition or legal prohibitions against ergogenic drugs. Dr. Robert Kerr equated ergogenic drug use with breast implants and plastic surgery, and argued that they should be freely available to anyone who wants to use scientific technology to augment their appearance, their performance, or their capacities. In Kerr's words, the athletes "are going to take them anyway," so legalization would ensure more thorough oversight of qualified medical professionals. Kerr's opinion does not reflect the dominant sports establishment, but it raises important questions: at what point does a supplement move from the realm of careful dietary and medical regulation of natural processes to an unnatural (and illegal) performance-enhancing drug? Both treatments are chemically based and both seek to improve the natural fitness and condition of an individual that does not take the supplements, so how are they distinguished?

All chemical supplements carry with them some level of side effects, so the distinction between natural and artificial cannot be based on safety alone. Kerr's argument suggests that such distinctions are imposed by certain metaphysical presumptions that assert human potential is defined by birth and that technological augmentation is unnatural. The advocates for legal ergogenic drugs argue that medical science always seeks to improve health and performance, and individuals should be permitted to take advantage of whatever technology provides. From this perspective, prohibiting ergogenic supplements is akin to denying the natural progress of technology.

On the other side, the advocates for strong anti-doping safeguards also often include moral arguments to support their position. In the introduction to Bob Goldman's influential book *Death in the Locker Room*, the inventor of the first commercially available steroid, John Ziegler, lamented that he "would never have imagined that the moral state of the sports world would change so dramatically." He recounted that when he started his medical practice in the 1940s, he found it difficult to convince the farmers to take a pill or receive an injection. Within his lifetime, "everything changed." The chemical revolution of the 1960s made everyone "pill happy." As Ziegler explained, because of the overreliance on chemical solutions, "not only are the athlete's lives in danger but that of our children and even the unborn." He called for public education campaigns to "bring some morality and sanity back to our athletic world."

At heart, the problem as Ziegler understood it was that society looked first to find an easy chemical solution for their weakness and only later thought about the consequences. This was echoed by the early enthusiasts for amateur sports. People like Pierre de Coubertin argued that sports promoted individual character by emphasizing teamwork and personal motivation. Winning was an outcome but not the primary objective of competition, which they viewed as an internal test of each athlete's pursuit of excellence. From this perspective, any drug that threatens individual health for the sake of external rewards is antithetical to the spirit of sport as a personal challenge. Moral values, such as discipline through individual restraint, perseverance despite adversity, and delayed gratification for the sake of higher objectives, can only emerge if victory in sport is viewed as a process rather than an exclusive objective. Ziegler's lament about the state of modern cultural and public morality reflects a fear that sport has been replaced by a new emerging culture that stresses chemical short cuts, personal excess, and victory at all costs.

Linking Anabolic Steroids and Catabolic Steroids

The public debates over the role of anabolic steroids more explicitly highlights the ambiguous position individuals sometimes find themselves as decision makers in determining suitable use options. For catabolic steroids, the culture places greater emphasis on individual priorities for determining the suitability of various therapeutic options rather than on legal regulations designed for consumer safety. In the case of anabolic steroids, the exact opposite is true—legal prohibitions reflect strong public pressure to restrict the individual's decision-making ability, and this presumption of consumer protection is so strong that it carries over into potential therapeutic options as well.

In both cases, however, the same fundamental question applies: does the short-term benefit of the steroid (whether anabolic or catabolic) exceed the long-term consequences of its use. Questions of competitive fairness not only seem to complicate this basic issue, but also rest on the presumption of a negative answer to the cost-benefit analysis. Though public consensus generally supports that conclusion, there remains room for some debate. In the next section, we consider how American society has determined the specific expectations of decision-making authority at the level of individual, public governance, and sports associations.

SECTION II

Contemporary Issues and Debates

CHAPTER 4

Individual Decision Making for Anabolic and Catabolic Steroids

When patients check into a hospital they usually receive a small pamphlet detailing their rights as an individual in determining their treatment and care. Every state includes a list of basic patient rights, and most states recommend that hospitals and clinics carry written notices of those rights. The Joint Commission of Illinois is one of the largest accrediting bodies for health care providers in the United States and their list of 14 rights that each patient should be made aware of includes:

1. The right to be informed about the care a patient will receive
2. The right to get information about the care in the language preferred by the patient
3. The right to receive information in a way that accommodates vision, speech, hearing, or mental impairments
4. The right to make decisions about a patient's care
5. The right to refuse care
6. The right to know the names of the caregivers who treat the patient
7. The right to safe care
8. The right to have pain addressed
9. The right to receive care free from discrimination
10. The right to know when something goes wrong with a patient's care
11. The right to obtain a list of all current medicines
12. The right to be listened to
13. The right to be treated with courtesy and respect
14. The right to have a personal representative (or advocate) present during care

In addition, each state includes numerous additional rights related to patient privacy and confidentiality. Finally, the federal government also mandates rights related to insurance, disclosure, and coverage. Most of these rights are detailed in written materials (like a pamphlet), and quite frequently, patients are asked to sign papers indicating that they have received and understand those rights.

The bulk of those rights can be summarized by a single principle: the individual has a right to make decisions about their health care. In terms of the therapeutic use of steroids for basic health care, the role and responsibility of the individual is no different than what would be expected for any other medical issue that affects a patient's health and well-being. For therapeutic decisions, patients are advised to use cost-benefit analysis to thoroughly consider expected benefits and potential risks of each medical treatment. When steroids are used for cosmetic or ergogenic purposes, then the expectations are more varied because the definitions by which we measure the cost or benefit may vary significantly according to the acceptable level of risk that each person is willing to tolerate. Ultimately, the individual is always responsible for decisions affecting personal health and well-being, whether those decisions are compelled by medical necessity or chosen through preference.

An individual's right to make informed medical decisions is often influenced by a variety of external factors that may have little to do with cost or benefits. Economic factors can play a significant role in limiting the number of options available to a patient. Likewise, marketing pressures may encourage patients to make decisions that are based on emotional rather than medical reasoning. Other factors, including a patient's age, their physical and psychological capacity may limit a patient's understanding of risks or benefits. These factors may greatly influence a patient's access to steroids, the licit and illicit pressures to use them, and their understanding of acceptable risk tolerance. The national discussion over the individual's role in choosing to use steroids includes a wide variety of opinions, and broad consensus is often difficult to find.

WHY INDIVIDUAL RIGHTS IN MEDICAL DECISION MAKING?

The importance of identifying individual patient rights is a reflection of the pace of scientific and technological development in medicine. Modern health care relies on highly specialized fields of scientific knowledge that are often limited to relatively few trained experts: doctors, nurses, and other health care practitioners. Most individuals do not have the expertise to make informed decisions for their personal health care, so they must rely on these experts. This may place patients in a vulnerable position of dependency, and there is a risk that the patient will blindly accept the recommendations of their doctor simply because they have no other basis for questioning their judgment.

The purpose behind legal policies emphasizing patients' rights is to ensure that both the individual and the doctor act in a voluntary relationship. The role of the doctor is to apply their expertise to the patient's unique situation, and the role of the patient is to consider that expertise or seek additional information elsewhere before making a final decision. Identifying specific rights helps protect both the patient and the doctor. The patient remains free to make decisions and the doctor is free to give responsible advice without enduring the burden of guaranteeing perfect results.

The rights of the individual, though, are not without limits. The natural scarcity of resources often forces individuals to forgo certain preferred health care options because of local availability of the doctor or technology, the inability to pay the costs of the specialized tools, or simply because the treatment is not accessible in the patient's geographic region. Likewise, the doctor is not always compelled to follow the patient's wishes. Sometimes, a patient may gain information about a treatment that the doctor does not deem effective or prudent, in which case the doctor is not necessarily bound to implement a treatment option that was not included in their initial recommendations. In these situations, the patient is free to go elsewhere. Moreover, the doctor is prohibited from implementing (much less recommending or suggesting) treatment options that are barred by law. In the case of illegal drugs or inappropriate applications of legal drugs (such as anabolic steroids for ergogenic purpose), both the rights of the doctor and the patient are restricted.

The concept of patient rights presumes that each individual is both bound and burdened by the freedom to make informed decisions about the own health care. If a patient chooses to follow a legal remedy that the doctor ordinarily provides, then the doctor must provide the care even if they disagree with the decision. At the same time, patients also may choose to be treated or not, even when it is clear that treatment might save their lives. That means each individual has a right to make an informed decision about their health care, even if that decision may prove detrimental to their overall well-being. These decisions will reflect the fundamental moral principles that each individual relies upon. In this way, individual medical decision making not only reflects civil rights, but most decisions also reflect larger cultural priorities.

DO ALL COUNTRIES RECOGNIZE INDIVIDUAL RIGHTS IN MEDICAL DECISION MAKING?

This is a good question. In most totalitarian societies, individuals have little to no say in how they are cared for or even whether they receive any kind of health care at all. Fortunately, in a civil society based on a presumption of democratic freedoms, each individual is encouraged to pursue their own personal, familial, or commercial relationships as they desire. The individual right to "life, liberty, and the pursuit of happiness" is a hallmark of American society, and those rights are assumed to belong to the individual first and are not bestowed by the government or collective society. As such, there must be some compelling justification for depriving an individual of their inherent right of determining the direction of their life or limiting their lawful pursuits. That is why individuals in free societies are given the primary responsibility for choosing how to pursue their health care options.

INFLUENCE OF HEALTH CARE INSURANCE

In a free society, we assume that individuals have the right to choose what they do to their bodies. For medical treatments, the right includes a presumption that the individual is making a free and informed decision before agreeing to a selected course of action. There are, however, a number of factors that influence or inhibit an individual's right to make such decisions freely or with adequate information.

Purpose of Health Insurance

In purely philosophical terms, each individual suffering from a disease should always be able to select from among all available options. In practical terms, though, the availability of some options is limited by financial expedience and resource availability. Certain procedures can be very expensive because they require highly specialized equipment run by highly trained people. Even though a given treatment option may significantly increase the possibility of extending a patient's life, if the treatment is scarce, the patient must compete with everyone else who shares the same diseases and some priority for access must be established. In non-free societies, those priorities are often determined by the government. In a free society, the access to certain donated resources is sometimes determined by need, time waiting, and other medical-based measures (such as for organ transplants). In other cases, where the resources are not donated, access is usually determined by a patient's ability to pay. We pay more for scarce treatments and less for treatments that are more easily available. Individual health insurance is intended to provide coverage for treatments that would otherwise be unavailable to a patient who has limited funds.

As with medical procedures, so too an individual's access to certain health insurance plans is limited by scarcity. Not all plans provide coverage for all ailments, and the availability of a particular plan depends on whether the patient is working or not, how much money their family earns, and whether their condition warrants long-term care (such as a disability or a preexisting condition). Depending on the size of the business, an employer may provide employees with a range of options to choose from, with varying costs reflecting different kinds of coverage depending on the employee's need (e.g., a single person may not need coverage for orthodontia). In some cases, the individual is presented with options, and then chooses the plan that best suits their needs.

The right to choose plans is often limited if an individual is not working or if their employer does not provide health insurance coverage. Most states provide subsidized health insurance plans depending on the patient's financial status, but government-based programs rarely include many plan options. In 2010, the U.S. Congress passed the Patient Protection and Affordable Care Act, which required all insurance companies to provide a certain minimum coverage of protection regardless of preexisting conditions of the patient. It also included a mandate requiring that all Americans must purchase insurance, either through their employer or through a state or federal government policy. The individuals maintained their right to choose options, but not their right to refuse coverage (without risk of financial penalty).

The Impact of Health Insurance on Individual Decision Making

The introduction of national health care mandates does not necessarily address the issue of resource scarcity. If a particular treatment is scarce and if priority is not regulated by a patient's ability to pay, the decision will inevitably revert to the insurance company—whether it is privately owned or administered through a state or federal government body. In cases of most catabolic steroids, scarcity is not a significant issue. Yet, even minor costs can be significant when multiplied by the millions of potential patients included in any given health insurance plan. In 1997, a study in the publication of *The Internet Journal of Anesthesiology* reviewed the use of corticosteroids (such as prednisone) as an anti-inflammatory agent during operations. Surgeons often administer glucocorticoids to patients on the presumption that the stress of the operation naturally inhibits the operation of the hypothalamic-pituitary-adrenal axis. The authors of the study concluded, "In the days of cost-conscious health care, the price of such testing will have to evaluated, while weighing the risks and benefits of such tests." The authors noted other side effects of the steroid supplement, including "delayed wound healing, increased susceptibility to infections, gastric ulcerations, catabolic effects on skin, muscle, bone and connective tissue and electrolyte disturbances." The significance is that the study indicated both economic and therapeutic considerations when evaluating the usefulness of the steroid treatment. There is some debate as to which consideration carries the greatest weight in determining the usefulness of any particular procedure: medical effectiveness or financial cost.

As medical costs increase, patients undergoing surgery may limit their options to those procedures that are covered by their insurance company. As insurance companies increase their role in such decisions (either as a result of public mandate requiring their involvement or as a result of unavoidable resource scarcity), then individual decision making becomes increasingly limited. Almost all insurance plans cover the prescription of catabolic steroids when used to address natural deficiencies caused by one or more pathologies of the endocrine system. The use of steroids as an anti-inflammatory is not as universal, however, since they address only the symptoms of the disorder and not the cause. In cases where the insurance plan does not cover the expenses, then the patient is forced to add the financial cost to their decision making. In some situations, this added cost eliminates the treatment as a viable option.

Insurance and the Debate between Elective and Therapeutic Treatments

Most insurance plans explicitly forbid the use of anabolic steroids for the purpose of performance enhancement. As a rule, any ergogenic drug would be excluded from coverage whether or not there is an explicit prohibition, because health insurance is limited to situations where the patient is suffering from an injury or disease—it is not generally used to cover elective lifestyle choices. There are some androgenic anabolic steroids that are covered by most insurance plans because they are part of a specific therapeutic treatment prescribed by a doctor (and not used for the purpose of performance enhancement). Some conditions where anabolic steroids may be prescribed include: AIDS wasting syndrome, anemia related to kidney failure, severe burns, weight loss due to cancer treatment, Klinefelter's syndrome, and other ailments resulting in a delayed growth or puberty. The purpose of the drug is usually critical in determining insurance coverage.

One of the most controversial exceptions to the rule of limiting insurance coverage to therapeutic treatments is birth control. Oral contraceptives are androgenic anabolic steroids that emphasize female sex characteristics rather than male sex characteristics. As such, they are not used for performance enhancement and are not included among the anabolic steroids listed in the Schedule III category of controlled substances by the Drug Enforcement Agency. There is considerable public debate as to whether oral contraceptives (or any form of artificial birth control) should be viewed as a therapeutic treatment or as an elective lifestyle choice. If birth control is a therapy, then conception and childbirth must be viewed as a pathology or as a biological disorder (rather than as an expression of health). Yet, if birth control is viewed as an elective lifestyle choice, then the long tradition of Title X public funding for family planning as a public health issue would have to be challenged. The political interests on both sides of the debate are magnified by divergent sets of core moral principles that are often mutually exclusive.

In 2012, Health and Human Services (HHS) secretary, Kathleen Sebalius, interpreted the 2010 Patient Protection and Affordable Care Act to mean that all insurance companies must provide coverage for all Food and Drug Administration (FDA)-approved birth control devices, including sterilization. Since the list of FDA-approved birth control measures include emergency contraceptives, which operate by destroying the ovum after fertilization (also known as an **abortifacient**), the HHS Mandate was opposed by a broad contingent of religious organizations, including Catholic hospitals and other faith-based institutions who may oppose artificial birth control, sterilization, or abortifacients on moral grounds. During the year following the decision, more than 200 plaintiffs filed 65 lawsuits challenging the constitutionality of the mandate. The issue was quickly politicized as part of the 2012 election, with the Democratic Party platform generally supporting the HHS mandate and the Republican Party platform generally opposing it. Political involvement transformed the issue into a cultural debate over moral and ideological norms.

As health insurance becomes the primary method for paying medical costs, the role of individual in decision making unavoidably decreases. The resulting cost-benefit analysis tends to place greater priority on economic considerations rather than on strict medical efficacy, which can trigger a great deal of public debate and controversy. Such debates only increase with state and federal government involvement through legal mandates and subsidies. Questions of whether a particular treatment is therapeutic or elective can easily become a forum for conflicting political interests rather than scientific assessment.

MARKETING PRESSURE FROM PHARMACEUTICAL INDUSTRIAL COMPLEX

Following the postwar biochemical revolution of the 1950s, the pharmaceutical industry developed marketing strategies that advertised medicines directly to the consumer. At that time, there were no federal regulations on drug labeling or advertising and the claims of pharmaceutical companies were not easily challenged. A worldwide scandal erupted in 1961, after doctors in more than 40 countries began prescribing thalidomide to pregnant women as a treatment for morning sickness, despite the fact that the drug was never approved for that indication. Reports of almost 10,000 cases of birth defects around the world (though not in the United States) prompted Congress to pass the Food, Drug and Cosmetic Act of 1962 granting the FDA authority to regulate drug labeling and advertising. The goal was to prevent the financial weight and vast marketing potential of the pharmaceutical companies from inappropriately influencing doctors and patients toward purchasing drugs that may not be medically necessary.

Advertising Guidelines

In 1969, the FDA established specific guidelines for advertisements that might reach the consumer directly (as opposed to marketing that targeted physicians). The guidelines included four criteria:

1. Advertisements must not contain false or misleading statements.
2. They must include a fair balance of risks and benefits.
3. They must only include facts that were materially relevant to approved uses.
4. They must include a brief summary of every known risk associated with the drug.

These conditions, particularly the fair balance and the brief summary requirements seemed too daunting for most drug manufacturers, who feared that the unvarnished description of risks might scare off an uninformed public. As a result, **direct-to-consumer** (DTC) marketing was very slow to reemerge. The first print advertisement for prescription drugs did not appear until 1981, when Merck purchased a full page ad in *Reader's Digest* for pneumovax (an antipneumococcal vaccine). It was another two years before a radio spot was broadcast for Rufen (a prescription version of the pain reliever, Motrin).

By the mid-1980s, drug manufacturers developed a partial solution to the fair balance and brief summary requirements through an advertising innovation, which relied on limited disclosure. They devised three kinds of DTC advertisements: (1) the "Help Seeking Ad," which provides information about a condition and a possible treatment with an encouragement for patients to contact their doctor for more information, but does not include the product name; (2) the "Reminder Ad," which includes the name of the product, information on its dosing, and pricing, but no mention of what it does or other claims of effectiveness; and (3) the "Product Claim Ad," which includes information about both product and its indications. Of the three options, the first two did not require the fair balance and brief summary components required by the FDA because neither makes any claims of effectiveness. For nearly a decade, pharmaceutical companies relied on limited print advertising for product claim ads, and used minimal radio and television spots to gain name brand recognition through help seeking and reminder ads. The broadcast mediums were impractical for product claim ads because air time was too expensive to sacrifice a significant proportion to the small print of the FDAs fair balance and brief summary requirements.

Advertising Reforms of 1997

The environment for DTC marketing of pharmaceutical products changed dramatically in 1997, when the FDA first published a draft of guidelines that significantly revised its requirements. Recognizing the limited time constraints of broadcast media, the FDA permitted drug companies to include a major statement of effectiveness followed by an adequate provision indicating risks, instead of the more extensive fair balance requirement. In addition, the FDA allowed a short list of major risks instead of the comprehensive brief summary requirement. These two changes made television and radio mediums much more viable as a conduit for marketing directly to consumers, and drug companies reacted immediately. The amount of money spent of DTC advertising rose from $12 million in 1980 to $47 million in 1990, to more than $788 million in 1997 and $1.2 billion the following year. By 2006, drug companies reached a zenith in spending with $5 billion devoted to DTC marketing. The subsequent economic recession triggered a decline in spending in the years that followed, but the overall expenditures still came close to $3.5 billion in 2013.

Scope of DTC Influence on Public Decision Making

The expanded marketing of the pharmaceutical industry had a major impact on the kinds of commercials people watched on a daily basis. By the 2010s, almost two-thirds of all DTC advertising was directed to television, with a little less than a third devoted to print media, and only about 5 percent committed to internet and other mass marketing techniques such as billboards and direct mailing.

Despite the onslaught of public advertising, the consumer did not necessarily increase overall public demand for medication. The new DTC approaches did not have any noticeable impact on the increasing rate of prescriptions filled in the United States. By 1990, the number of scripts written was already coming very near to the two billion mark. A decade later in 2000 that number had increased to nearly three billion, and by the following decade in 2010, the total had reached almost four billion (which is a little more than a dozen per person). The major pivot point in DTC advertising came in the late 1990s, yet the rate of increase (1 billion per decade) was unchanged between 1990, 2000, and 2010. Nevertheless, the DTC marketing did have a significant impact on brand name recognition, and that change occurred very quickly. By 1999, doctors were writing 34 percent more prescriptions for the drugs that were being advertised by DTC, compared to the 5 percent increase in prescriptions written overall. By 2001, doctors reported a significant increase in the annual number of patients requesting at least one brand name prescription.

DOES DIRECT-TO-CONSUMER ADVERTISING WORK?

Contrary to common intuition, the amount of money spent advertising a drug does not necessarily result in equivalent changes in sales or popularity. In 2012, the five top advertised drugs were Cymbalta (at $243 million), Embrel (at $168 million), Cialis (at $162 million), Humira (at $141 million), and Celebrix (at $129 million). Yet, only two of those were listed among the five top selling drugs: Humira reaped $9.48 billion and Embrel grossed $8.37 billion. Cymbalta ranked among the top 15 top selling drugs (at $5 billion), but Celebrix and Cialis did not. In part, the difference between advertisement and global sales reflects the fact that only the United States and New Zealand allow DTC advertising, which means that elsewhere in the industrialized world, most prescriptions are based on doctor recommendation only and not consumer request. In part, also, the difference reflects the fact that some treatments are so specialized that patients rarely feel empowered enough to request them. For example, 4 of the top 15 selling prescription drugs are for cancer-related treatments used in chemotherapy: Rituxan (at $7.67 billion), Herceptin (at $6.08 billion), Avastin (at $5.98 billion), and Gleevec (at $4.72 billion).

Typically, pharmaceutical companies devote most of their DTC marketing budgets to drugs that may potentially be requested by patients. Many of these drugs involve lifestyle issues (such as erectile dysfunction or artificial contraceptives) or involve treatments for chronic illnesses (such as allergies, asthma, high cholesterol, or depression). For either situation, a patient might change treatment options several times during their lifetime. The degree to which DTC marketing might influence individual patient decision making is often based on a corresponding sense of urgency of need. In this context, catabolic steroids used to treat asthma are most likely to be influenced by DTC advertising. For example, in 2012, $99 million was spent advertising Advair (resulting in $8 billion return). Yet, other catabolic steroids used for presurgery preparations or other treatments used for unique endocrine deficiencies were mostly left off the DTC budgets. That does not mean they are not marketed—instead, the advertising was directed exclusively to the physician. As a ratio of total marketing budgets, DTC advertising remains a little more than half of what was spent advertising directly to physician. In the end, doctor recommendation remained the strongest basis for determining drug sales.

Public Controversy over DTC Marketing

In terms of the impact on individual decision making, there are arguments that support and oppose the significant increase in DTC marketing. Opponents argue that the barrage of emotionally charged images transmitted to underinformed consumers leads to artificial demands for chemical solutions for ordinary problems, or to unrealistic expectations of positive results from drugs that may have only limited indications. By 2011, the average viewer could count on watching at least nine drug-related television commercials per day, adding up to 16 hours of exposure per year, which is more time than most people spend with their primary care physician. Critics argue that drug companies are interposing themselves between patient and physician, which may result in misdiagnosis or self-diagnosis for ailments that have more complicated solutions.

By contrast, supporters contend that DTC marketing empowers patients with options that they may not otherwise be aware of. The advertisements encourage patients to contact their physicians more regularly, and promote dialog between the patient and physician during situations when the patient may otherwise simply defer to the first treatment option offered to them. Also, supporters argue that those emotionally charged images can have a positive effect by removing the stigma of certain diseases or ailments that people may otherwise be too embarrassed to bring up to their doctor, such as erectile dysfunction or depression. Moreover, since all prescriptions

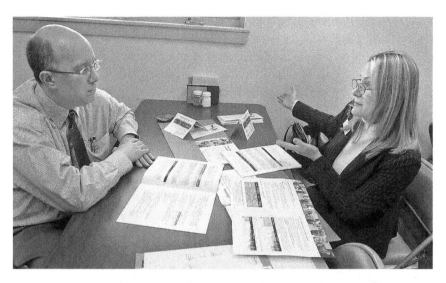

Drug information consultant Leigh Bradshaw of Independent Drug Information Service talks with Dr. Ernest Josef at his Pennsylvania practice in 2008. Pennsylvania is among a handful of states trying to counter the pharmaceutical industry's multibillion-dollar marketing and cut costs for prescription-aid programs for senior citizens, who are bombarded with "ask your doctor" advertising. (AP Photo/Jason Minick)

must still be written by the doctor, the DTC advertising has no effect on the doctor's role as gatekeeper for potentially dangerous drugs.

DTC Advertising of Anabolic Steroids

The public debate over the impact of DTC advertising is more lopsided when it comes to potentially nontherapeutic uses of prescription drugs. Of particular concern is the prospect that drug companies might use their advertising skills to exploit popular cultural insecurities to stimulate public support for pathologies that do not exist in strictly scientific terms. For example, there is some debate in the medical community as to whether low testosterone is a legitimate ailment for aging men. Testosterone levels naturally begin to taper off as men reach later middle age. The desire to find a magical antiaging pill is very high in a culture that is so heavily influenced by an aging Baby Boom population. Emotionally charged television commercials that play off the natural anxieties related to old age may be sufficient to create a demand for legal anabolic steroids, by marketing them as testosterone replacement therapies.

In 2012, the pharmaceutical industry made $2 billion in such legal sales of androgenic anabolic steroids that were marketed for therapeutic use. Yet, there is little consensus within the medical community as to whether the benefits of supplemental testosterone in older men outweighs the potential side effects. As the various physiological systems in the body begin to enter new phases following middle age, there is an increased risk that continual addition of youth-related sex hormones may lead to unintended health risks. Critics argue that DTC advertising applies inappropriate pressure on underinformed patients to pursue treatments for manufactured ailments, which in turn pressures doctors to reframe their definitions of medical necessity. In such cases, the individual would be making judgments that effect their individual health and well-being based on the economic interests of the drug industry rather than on the merits of scientific evidence.

The Influence of DTC Marketing on Cultural Priorities

Much of the criticism leveled at DTC advertising (whether for testosterone or for other potentially voluntary drug treatments) reflect deeper moral and philosophical issues. A common theme among arguments against television advertising for such treatments as artificial contraceptives, weight loss, erectile dysfunction, and depression is that they seem to promise a chemical-based solution for problems that may be social in nature. The moral controversies associated with promoting artificial contraceptives are better discussed elsewhere, but the core conflict most often stems from moral presumptions about appropriate behaviors—a pill will not eliminate the emotional and physical consequences that accompany risky sexual behaviors. Similarly, weight loss may be accelerated through the use of certain drugs, but most lasting results require significant lifestyle changes. Erectile dysfunction and depression can be evaluated in the same manner. Critics argue that the routine exposure to chemical solutions reinforces an unrealistic cultural expectation of instant gratification and easy solutions. Such attitudes discourage the necessary characteristics that truly define individual empowerment. In this context, the increase of DTC marketing potentially restricts individual decision making, because it leads to habitual and misinformed choices rather than free and informed decisions.

OTHERS FACTORS LIMITING INDIVIDUAL DECISION MAKING

Others factors related to a patient's ability to understand their conditions or their treatment options invariably influence or inhibit an individual's right to make an informed decision. Very young children, patients who are not conscious (through illness or trauma), and those with psychological conditions that limit their systematic reasoning abilities must rely on advocates to act on their behalf in medical decision making. In some cases, the patient may retain the use of their reasoning faculties, but may still defer to nonmedical advocates for their health care decisions.

Obligations and Limitations of Parental Rights in Medical Decisions

In the case of infants, toddlers, and adolescents, the doctor usually assumes the health care decisions are determined by the parent or a legal guardian. This is based on legal precedents derived from the First Amendment protections of speech and religious expression. Each parent has a right to raise their child in a way they deem most appropriate. These parental rights are framed by legal obligations to care for children and to refrain from action that might endanger the children's physical or mental health. In terms of medical decision making, all decisions may potentially have an impact on a child's health, so the presumption of parental obligations revolve around questions of potential harm or aid to the child. If a parent demonstrates an inability to make proper decisions for the well-being of the child—either for mental or physical reasons—or if the parent appears unwilling to make such decisions, then the state may intervene and assume custody.

The state must presume parental jurisdiction and must assume the burden of proving that parents have failed in their obligations (medical neglect) before it can claim legal guardianship. The burden is high, and usually the state does not get involved unless the consequences of inaction involve situations that threaten the life of the child. Common examples include parents, who for religious reasons, choose to withhold treatment for their children. In such cases, the state must prove that the expected benefits of treatment were significantly greater than the risks of no treatment, and further that potential alternatives were more detrimental than the traditionally prescribed course. In 1991, the Supreme Court decided in *Newmark v. Williams* that the decision of Christian Scientist parents to withhold chemotherapy treatment for their son's diagnosis of Burkitt's lymphoma was justified because the treatment only promised a 40 percent chance of success and involved significant toxic side effects. If the treatment guaranteed greater than 50/50 chance of success, then the court could have compelled the parents to act because the consequences of inaction was probable death.

For most other nonlife-threatening decisions, the parents usually maintain primary responsibility. For example, procedures to repair a cleft palate or to circumcise a male child result in permanent consequences for the child, but they do not endanger the physical or mental health of the child, and so the decisions rest entirely with the parents. There are, however, situations when withholding treatment for nonreligious reasons may lead to charges of medical neglect, even if the treatment does not involve life or death consequences. In an Oklahoma case, *In the Matter of D.R.* (2001), the Court of Appeals ruled that parents who withheld physical therapy for their child who suffered seizures and developmental difficulties were neglecting the needs of the child, even though the parents believed the physical therapy was responsible for the seizures. The court relied on the recognized authority of medical experts who provided evidence that continued treatment would substantially improve the health and well-being of the child. In order to reject the advice of accepted medical practice, the parents would have had to provide a suitable alternative that promised at least comparable chances of successful treatment. Since the parents had no religious objection to the physical therapy, then the court ordered the parents to resume treatment for their child.

ORAL CONTRACEPTION EXCEPTION

While the courts recognizes the primacy of parental rights in their child's medical decision making in most cases involving therapeutic treatment options, many states carved out special exceptions for anabolic steroids used for oral contraceptives. In 2010, 26 states and the District of Columbia passed legislation allowing minors 12 and older to receive contraceptives without the need of parental approval. An additional 20 states allow only certain categories of minors to receive such services and only 4 states have no laws governing the matter. The public usually does not think of oral contraceptives as an anabolic steroid, and the debate over whether they are therapeutic or nontherapeutic is strongly tied to larger moral, political, and economic debates. In these cases, medical considerations were less influential than ideological considerations.

Influence of Nontraditional Medicine on Parental Decision Making

In most cases involving questions of steroid use, there are few religious objections and they rarely involve situations of life or death. Nevertheless, there is always potential for an alternative therapy involving steroid hormones as a treatment for serious diseases. Nontraditional medicine does not rely on scientific methodology to demonstrate effectiveness. For example, some people place great faith in laetrile as a popular alternative to chemotherapy for cancer fighting. Sometimes referred to a vitamin B_{17}, laetrile is a nonhormonal steroid (glycoside) molecule that is derived from the seeds of apricots, peaches, or almonds. The use of bitter almonds to treat serious illnesses dates back to preindustrial times in regions such as China, Egypt, and among the Pueblo Indians, but modern interest grew out of anecdotal stories pointing to very low cancer rates in certain central Asian cultures. The populations living along India's northern border eat diets rich in laetrile, and the treatment emerged in the United States among those seeking alternatives to western medicine.

Two cases emerged during the late 1970s in New York and Massachusetts, where parents were charged with medical neglect for withholding traditional chemotherapy in favor of nontraditional remedies. In both cases, parents refused treatment for their children suffering from blood cancers, and instead pursued nontraditional treatments based around the steroid laetrile. In one case, the court allowed the parents to continue the laetrile treatments provided it was supervised by a licensed physician, and in the other, the court ordered the parents to treat their child with traditional chemotherapy. There are no studies that demonstrate evidence that laetrile has any potential for successfully treating cancer, and there are several studies that indicate high toxic effects.

In 1977, the FDA recommended legal prohibitions against the sale or transport of laetrile because of its potential for abuse among those seeking alternative remedies. Laetrile interacts with other glycosides to release cyanide into the system, and most states have outlawed its use due to clinical studies pointing to cyanide poisoning. Nevertheless, as late as the 2010s, numerous articles were found online touting laetrile as a miracle cure, and the drug may be purchased through numerous websites inside and outside the United States.

The popularity of a drug treatment is sometimes based more on anecdotal rather than scientific evidence, and the future priorities of nontraditional therapies are not easy to predict. Potentially, any number of hormone-based anabolic and catabolic steroids could be repurposed as a fashionable alternative to traditional therapy because they play such a significant role in the endocrine system. The likelihood for this is much stronger for anabolic steroids due to the significant illicit use and trafficking of the drugs for ergogenic purposes. When individuals self-medicate and illegally use prescription drugs outside the oversight of a doctor, then there is a much greater likelihood for urban legends to replace scientific methodology for treatment options. The prospect of nontraditional alternatives may be especially appealing to parents of children suffering from life-threatening diseases, who reach out to unconventional sources in the hope of finding potential cures. In such cases, the decisions made on a child's behalf may be freely undertaken, but may still be based on questionable information.

Criteria for Determining Need for Legal Guardianship or Legal Advocate

Parents are automatically presumed to be the primary advocate for their children's health care decisions. Once a young adult reaches the age of maturity, parents no longer act automatically as their advocates. In some states, the age at which a child can make medical decisions is lower than the traditional majority. For example, in Virginia, the age is 14 years for some types of decisions that do not involve life-threatening options. Yet, even when a child reaches adulthood, they may still choose to rely on their parent's recommendations in health care decisions. In such cases, the parents act as their children's advocate and not as their guardian.

Any adult may choose an advocate for any number of reasons that may have as much to do with emotional comfort as it does with their capacity to make informed decisions. A husband may choose to bring his wife to a medical consultation because he trusts her opinion, or an elderly parent may choose to bring their adult child, or a patient may bring a close friend for similar reasons. In these cases, the advocacy is informal and the doctor respects their presence in the consultation because it reflects the wish of the patient.

In other cases, advocacy may be based on a more formal need. If an adult patient suffers from a psychological or physiological disorder that limits their reasoning abilities, then the doctor may request that a responsible advocate be present to help in the decision-making process. For example, a patient suffering from age-related dementia or from a neurological trauma (such as a stroke or an accident) may require the help of an advocate to help them engage in informed decision making. Formal determination of competency is left to the court system, but a doctor may make informal recommendations.

The criteria for determining an adult's competency to make health-related decisions are based on four variables: (1) Does the patient acknowledge relevant information? (2) Do they appreciate the circumstances of their condition? (3) Do they make logical use of information? (4) Can they communicate their choices? Patients acknowledge relevant information when they remember relevant facts related to their condition and are aware of their role in the decision-making process. Additionally, they should show that they understand the importance of different treatment options, including both short-term benefits and potential long-term risks. Most importantly, patients should be able to provide reasonable explanations for their eventual decisions, and then be able to communicate those preferences consistently over time. Failure to demonstrate these cognitive tasks may indicate that the patient is not capable of engaging in free and informed decisions about their health care without some help from a formal or informal advocate.

Influence of Informal Advocates

The responsibilities of both formal and informal advocates are similar to those carried by parents for their children's medical health. Advocates are expected to make decisions that ensure that any potential benefits outweigh the possible health risks. There are moral and legal presumptions that guard against advocates making decisions that expose their charges to unnecessary risks.

For most cases, informal advocates are friends or loved ones chosen by the patient directly and there is little risk that they would deliberately encourage the patient to pursue treatments that may lead to inappropriate risks. This is especially true when the medical questions involve therapeutic options. There are some cases, however, when this presumption is tested (such as between an athlete and their coach or personal trainer), where a patient may rely on an advocate for medical advice outside the doctor's office and for purposes unrelated to general health. The medical questions that arise from such relationships usually involve performance enhancement, and the ultimate objective of long-term health may not be the primary priority for either the patient or the advocate.

Not infrequently, athletes who test positive for ergogenic drugs claim that they did not know they were taking steroids. During the Beijing Olympics in 2008, Ukrainian heptathlon silver medalist Lyudmila Blonska was stripped of her medal and banned from competition for life after failing a drug test, which indicated she had taken methyltestosterone. She later blamed her coach/husband for the doping because she had trusted him to be responsible for her training and her diet. Similarly, in 2013, Ultimate Fighting Championship light heavyweight fighter Joey Beltran was drug tested following his fight with Igor Pokrajac. He tested positive and was suspended for nine months for using Nandrolone. Beltran also claimed he did not take the steroid, but admitted that he may have received the drug from his trainer who told him he was taking a dietary supplement. In both situations, the anti-doping authorities did not care whether the athletes knowingly took the drug or not and the suspension remained in effect.

For therapeutic treatments, the patient rarely worries about the legality of the treatment. A prescription from a recognized, licensed physician is often all that is needed to transform a controlled substance into a legal therapy. It is conceivable that a patient might receive a prescription, have it filled by a pharmacist, and take the recommended doses without fully knowing what kind the drug is or what the expected side effects will be. Yet, the decision to accept the treatment remains free and informed because it rests on an implicit trust in the doctor's technical knowledge.

The legal and procedural safeguards that are set in place to build up such trust do not carry over to the relationship between patient and informal advocate. Individuals who willingly abdicate their decision-making responsibilities to an informal advocate who may place competitive goals ahead of medical safety, runs a risk of inappropriate advocacy. That risk is especially high when the treatments involve anabolic steroids or other ergogenic drugs that may or may not be legally sanctioned by civil authorities.

CONCLUSION

The difference between responsibly using steroids for therapeutic use, and irresponsibly abusing them for ergogenic or recreational use depends on the motivation of the individual choosing to use them. When prescribed by a licensed physician to treat a specific ailment, any drug (including both catabolic and anabolic steroid types) may be used for therapeutic purposes. The decision to use the recommended therapy or to follow the recommended treatment schedule rests with the individual. With the exception of parental rights or legal advocates for adults with impaired decision-making faculties, each individual patient maintains first responsibility for their health care decisions. In a free society, this responsibility is protected. Certain practical economic, cultural, and ethical considerations will inevitably limit the available options, but the responsibility to make a free and informed decision about medical treatment remains a philosophical and legal right.

Most controversies regarding medical decisions arises when the individual chooses medical solutions from sources outside the auspices of a licensed physician, or when the individual gives up that right to someone else who may choose to make decisions outside the traditional medical establishment. A parent's right to determine the health care options of their children are rarely questioned, except in those circumstances when they pursue treatments that are not broadly recognized by the medical community. An advocates' influence over their charge only becomes suspect when it involves recommendations that are made in isolation of recognized medical authorities. The definition of abuse usually involves using potentially hazardous drugs for purposes that are not recognized as therapeutic.

When individuals make medical decisions that impact people other than themselves, then the civil authorities usually step in to establish guidelines. Legal regulations regarding parental rights and formally recognized advocates for impaired adults attempt to preserve the basic principle of individual decision making. Parents and advocates are given the right to choose medical options based on free and informed decisions. At the same time, if there is evidence that the resulting decisions are not well informed based on the standards established by the medical establishment, then the civil authorities may intervene. Yet, in such cases, the state intervention must still adhere to the principle of respecting the wishes and preferences of the protected individual.

For the most part, these issues rarely arise from the use of catabolic steroids that are almost always used for therapeutic purposes. By contrast, the use of anabolic steroids is highly susceptible to challenges from civil authorities, because they are most likely to be abused as an ergogenic drug. Economic and cultural trends influence the medical community in their evaluation of the long-term health risks of anabolic steroids. The degree to which the public demands legal prohibition invariably reflects cultural priorities that are often flexible, and reflect specific historical events. In the next chapter, we consider the ideology behind the role of civil authorities in educating (and compelling) individual decision making with regard to anabolic steroids.

CHAPTER 5

Public Reaction, Regulation, and Control

In a civil society, the state regulates practices that are deemed by popular consensus to be disruptive to the general welfare of the population. In an effort to protect the innocent from the harmful actions of others, lawmakers draft laws that prohibit certain practices through legal sanction. Some crimes are obvious by their very nature (called *mala in se*), and include acts of violence, theft, and deception. Other crimes are only so because society has determined them to be so (called *mala prohibita*), and these might include smoking or driving too fast on a highway. Public controversies over legalization or criminalization most often concern those practices that are not universally recognized as disruptive. In many cases, debates over criminalization reflect deep moral differences over the relative value of individual restraint versus free action.

Public consensus over moral norms often changes over time. In 1930, gambling was illegal, the sale and manufacturing of alcohol was illegal, as were most judgment-impairing drugs—such as marijuana. A little more than 80 years later, after the 2012 elections, legal gambling can be found in every state, the consumption of alcohol is legal for adults aged 21 years or older, and two states have decriminalized marijuana use for recreational purposes. Public consensus on the relative dangers to self and society associated with each activity has changed over time, as a reflection of changing standards of what constitutes personal health and acceptable risk. In the 1920s, moral health was considered to be just as important as physical health. In the 2010s, questions of morality are rarely introduced into the public forum. Most public policy debates focus on practical cost-benefit assessments of potential dangers to physical, psychological, and emotional health. The immaterial values of individual or public morality are rarely vocalized in the discussion of decriminalization—though they may often play a deciding role in eventual public support.

Such practical reasoning was notable during the 2012 election cycle, which included ballot measures in three states seeking to legalize marijuana for recreational use. The arguments against legalization faced an uphill battle because the question was largely framed in terms of immediate risks to personal health and community. In earlier eras, the debate would have included commonly accepted moral values, such as individual moral restraint, sobriety for unobstructed judgment, positive public modeling, and the need to protect the character development of youth. In 2012, the debate concentrated on whether marijuana posed a greater health risk than other legally available substances (mainly alcohol), and whether decriminalization would free up resources that were ordinarily used for police and prosecution. Absent from the public forum were any judgments about whether pot smoking was morally wrong, if it contributed to unhealthy cultural priorities, or if it led to immoral behaviors. The dominant focus on the presence (or absence) of immediate risks made arguments about long-term consequences or corruption of intangible values less compelling. After the election, sizable majorities in two of the three states (Colorado and Washington) approved the ballot measures.

Similar debates confront the question of legalizing anabolic steroids for competitive or recreational use. The potential for either side capturing public support is based largely on whether the question is framed in terms of short-term dangers or long-term consequences. Like marijuana, the immediate consequences of steroid use for ergogenic purposes are not always apparent. There are certainly very famous cases of illness and deaths during competition related to doping, but they are fairly rare and most athletes caught using steroids show no immediate health risks. In the long term, the physical and psychological dangers of steroid abuse are much easier to demonstrate but the prospect that any individual athlete will experience those consequences is still based on probabilities. If the debate is focused only on immediate practical material consequences, then there is little defense against arguments for legalization. But, if the argument includes long-term consequences and moral considerations, then arguments for criminalization tend to have a stronger case.

Both sides of the legalization debate reflect differing presuppositions about moral reasoning, so each is vulnerable to legitimate challenges from those who do not share the same priorities. Though public consensus continues to support legal prohibitions, history provides ample evidence that such priorities are liable to change. Whether or not anabolic steroids will continue to face legal sanctions will depend upon how the public chooses to measure individual health risks and its associated cultural disruptions.

LIMITATIONS TO INDIVIDUAL DECISION MAKING

If a civil society guarantees certain individual liberties (the right to pursue happiness in their own way), why would the right of an individual to consume any form of drug ever be challenged? If the drugs are ingested individually and voluntarily, then why should the individual not be allowed to enjoy (or suffer) whatever consequences there may be as a reflection of their decision making? If individual drug use for nontherapeutic purposes affects no one but the individual, then why should civil government regulate the activity? Such questions reflect purely practical considerations, and their answers usually involve a consideration of less-obvious factors such as the individual's latent impact on society and the costs of an individual's absence from society.

In terms of an individual's impact on society, the role of the individual in medical care decision making is largely determined by the degree by which those decisions harm others or themselves. In cases of medical necessity (therapeutic uses), the primary authority for judging whether the desired benefits outweigh the anticipated risks of a treatment is left to the individual patient. In such cases, the patient is already afflicted with an ailment, so the social costs of treating the ailment are generally recognized as less severe than the costs of leaving it alone. The unalienable rights of individual liberty guarantee the individual's primary authority to make therapeutic decisions. In most cases where catabolic steroids are at question, this standard applies.

In cases of elective procedures, individual liberty is shared by those others that might also be affected by the patient's decisions. If any voluntary drug treatment carries a high risk of impacting society at large, then the civil authorities must be included, usually resulting in legal regulations. For example, cocaine promotes aggressive behaviors and is so addictive that users often resort to crime to pay for their habit. Individuals do not have the sole authority to determine whether or not they want to assume the risks of ingesting cocaine. The government denies individuals the right to use cocaine because there is very little therapeutic value in the drug and because the social impact of cocaine addiction poses too great a risk of harming other members of the society, including family, friends, and community. Additionally, cocaine use impairs an individual's ability to be a productive member of the society, so even if the effects of the drug could be completely restricted to the individual alone, the society would be deprived of the individual's contribution.

Noncompetitive Uses—Recreation or Cosmetic Choice

The same logic follows for drugs that may impact select individuals, though perhaps not society at large. In such cases, the association of those people most likely to be effected by the drug use must also be included in the decision-making process before the individual can take the drug. For example, if an athlete competing in a sports event takes performance-enhancing drugs, then his actions affect the other competitors who must face a more difficult challenge as a result of the drug. Depending on the potency of the drug, the practical effects of performance enhancement may or may not impact society at large. The decision to regulate, then, is sometimes left to the effected group (e.g., the sports association that organized the competitive event) and does not necessarily mandate government intervention. This is why some performance-enhancing drugs, such as the steroid precursor androstenedione is prohibited for professional baseball players but is legal for an amateur softball player.

Public controversy usually arises when the ergogenic drugs are used not only for noncompetitive purposes, but also for nontherapeutic use. For example, if an aging man wants to regain his youthful physique, then how would his decisions to risk the side effects of a testosterone supplement affect society at large? Public debate over recreational or cosmetic use of anabolic steroids focuses on whether the drugs pose any significant risk to society. If the only people to be effected are other competitors in the sports community, why should the government get involved through legal prohibitions? If the basis of decision making is purely pragmatic, then those supporting criminalization (to limit the individual's authority to make their own judgments about the level of acceptable risk) must assume the burden of showing that the drugs pose significant and measurable physical risks to society. If the decision making includes moral factors, then the potential risk need not be as quantifiable.

TRIGGERS OF GOVERNMENT INVOLVEMENT

Most people recognize the potential dangers that would threaten society if hard drugs like cocaine or heroin were legalized for recreational use. The difficulty arises when the discussion involves drugs with less obvious health risks. Prolonged use of androgenic anabolic steroids have been shown to lead to serious health risks, but the effects of limited use are not as obvious and causal evidence remains elusive. At what point do prospective risks to society require government involvement to prohibit the drug? In theory, modern lawmakers rely exclusively on arguments that balance the prospective benefits against the potential risks to physical and psychological health to make these decisions. In actual practice, the deeper underlying justifications may rely on less tangible explanations.

Clinical Evidence of Health Risks

The Centers for Disease Control and Prevention (CDC) provides a long list of clinical studies that show significant correlation between the use of anabolic steroids and increased risks for liver damage and liver tumors, higher blood pressure, decreased myocardial (heart related) functioning, and other cancers. Additionally, there is considerable anecdotal evidence of 20–25-year-old weightlifters dropping dead from myocardial infarctions (heart attacks) during the course of their training regimen. Postmortem autopsies reveal very high levels of androgenic anabolic steroids in their system. Ordinarily, 20–25-year-olds in good health do not suffer such ailments, so it is easy to conclude that the steroid use is what triggered the attacks. When these news items are combined with other more sensational news stories about elite athletes dying during their competitions, such as cyclists Knud Jensen and Tom Simpson, it is easy to conclude that all ergogenic drugs—anabolic steroids, especially—pose serious health risks.

In fact, there are no clinical studies that show a direct causal connection between anabolic steroid use and myocardial infarctions or cancer growth. In a 2006 article in the *Journal of Sports Science and Medicine*, Jay R. Hoffman and Nicholas A. Ratamess reviewed existing research and confirmed that there is a relationship between users and increased rates of risk—but there is no way to be certain that the increased risks are not due to some other agent or to some combination of factors that may or may not be directly tied to anabolic steroid use. Genetic predisposition, diet, or other environmental factors may pose greater risks than the steroids. The quantifiable evidence is not sufficient to make a final determination. The absence of clinical evidence does not mean that such causal relationships do not exist—it only means that there is not enough evidence to be certain one way or another.

If we set aside issues of competitive fairness, and if we also exclude the more traditional ideals associated with natural (unaided) physical fitness, then why are anabolic steroids for performance enhancement illegal? What kinds of health risks do anabolic steroids pose to the larger society that requires legal prohibition? The range of side effects that appear with enough regularity to assume some causal connection are not necessarily life threatening nor do they necessarily impact others. Acne, male pattern baldness, deepening of the voice, testicular shrinkage and low sperm counts for men, gynecomastia and facial hair for women, libido changes, and menstrual irregularities are all sufficiently demonstrable to suggest a causal relationship with anabolic steroid use. Yet, none of these physical ailments necessarily threaten life expectancy, and in most cases they are not likely to result in permanent changes. Advocates for legalization of anabolic steroids argue that these health risks have minimal impact on society, and each individual should be allowed to determine their own threshold of acceptable risk.

Less Quantifiable Health Risks—Roid Rage

Opponents of legalization of anabolic steroids argue that there are other psychological risks that are more difficult to measure, but nevertheless pose far greater risks to society. Beginning in the 1980s, numerous studies demonstrated strong correlations between anabolic steroid use and increased aggressiveness, irritability, and mood swings. One study indicated 60 percent of users experienced these effects, and another nationwide survey showed that users were much more likely than nonusers to report engaging in acts of violence against people or causing damage to property resulting from outbursts of aggression. Another study examined the testimonies of 41 steroid users and found that 22 percent exhibited manic or depressive behaviors and 12 percent experienced psychotic episodes. These clinical studies accompanied a host of other anecdotal accounts of bodybuilders and weightlifters suffering from extreme mood swings, leading to uncontrollable outbursts of violence. By the early 1990s, the phrase "roid rage" could be found in almost any book dealing with anabolic steroids—regardless of whether the information was intended to support or oppose their legal use.

As was the case with physical health risks, the causal connection between anabolic steroid use and roid rage has not been definitively established. Yet, the correlational evidence is strong. In an article from the *Archives of General Psychology*, researchers in Sweden studying inmates at local jails and drug treatment centers found that steroid users were twice as likely to have been convicted of weapons offenses than was the general population. In 2008, another nationwide survey confirmed the earlier 1980s study, and found that adolescents who admitted to using steroids were also more likely to admit to aggressive and violent behaviors. The popular presumption of roid rage is so common that defense attorneys occasionally use it as a form of insanity defense for their client's violent behaviors. Horace Williams was accused of killing a hitchhiker in Florida in 1988 and his attorney claimed Williams's use of anabolic steroids for competitive bodybuilding led to a temporary drug-induced episode at the time of the killing. The defense strategy was not successful and Williams was convicted, but other attorneys have successfully argued diminished capacity due to steroid use to help reduce the sentence after conviction. The perception among users and observers of violence provides a popular justification for arguing that anabolic steroids create an unnecessary hazard to the public health.

The problem with establishing a direct causal connection between anabolic steroids and uncontrollable outbursts of violence is that the people most likely to use the ergogenic drugs are also the kinds of people that are most likely to be engaged in a routinely competitive lifestyle. Athletes are often trained to channel their aggressive tendencies to hone their competitive edge. In some cases, coaches and trainers encourage their athletes to use emotional imagery as a concentration aid for overcoming the physical and emotional pains that go along with fierce competition. It is difficult for researchers to separate the aggressive tendencies associated with intense training from those tendencies that are chemically induced by anabolic steroids. One study in 2004 examined a group of nonathletes who were given testosterone injections over a 10-week period unaccompanied by a fitness routine of diet and exercise. The researcher concluded that the testosterone by itself did not elevate aggressive behaviors. While this single study is not sufficient to overcome the other correlational studies, it does suggest that the association between anabolic steroids use and psychological outbursts is more complicated than a singular biochemical interaction.

Parallel Risk Levels: Alcohol, Marijuana, and Anabolic Steroids

The difficulty with demonstrating the physical and psychological risks of anabolic steroids is similar to the tasks of demonstrating the medical hazards of recreational marijuana use. In both cases, the immediate health risks appear to be minimal for initial or limited use.

Marijuana users experience increased heart rates, impaired coordination and reflexes, and a distorted sense of time and space often resulting in problems with short-term memory and learning. The high that someone experiences while under the influence of marijuana is due to the delta-9-tetrahydrocannabinol (**THC**) molecule interaction overstimulating the cannabinoid receptors in the brain that trigger an elevated sense of pleasure. It also affects memory, concentration, critical thinking, and sensory perception, which accounts for the sense of distorted reality. In many cases, the symptoms of the drug interaction may appear similar to alcohol-related intoxication, but the causes are different. Alcohol inhibits certain neurotransmitters (glutamate), which results in a slowdown of the electrical impulses of the brain. It also stimulates the production of dopamine which creates the sense of pleasure associated with drinking. By contrast, THC stimulates receptor reactions.

One of the differences between marijuana use and alcohol use is the range of physical symptoms that become manifest between mild and heavy use, particularly the distorted sense of reality that follows consumption. The spectrum of physical symptoms that follow alcohol consumption can range broadly from little to no effect to an incapacitating effect. By contrast, the physical symptoms of marijuana are more narrowly constrained. At its most extreme range, high blood alcohol levels can suppress the central nervous system leading to a loss of consciousness or death, while heavy consumption of marijuana will result in loss of coordination and motor control but will rarely lead to physiological shut down. At the opposite end of the spectrum, small amounts of alcohol will have little impact on perception, while even small amounts of THC will stimulate the cannabinoid receptors and alter the user's sense of reality. In part, the differences have to do with the method of delivery—alcohol can be consumed in a variety of concentrations, whereas THC is conveyed through marijuana smoke in limited doses. More intense concentrations of THC would certainly result in a similarly broad range of symptoms.

It is popular to say that marijuana is harmless because no one has ever died from the drug. That is not actually true. The Food and Drug Administration (FDA) recorded 279 deaths between 1997 and 2005 linked to marijuana abuse, and 187 deaths were attributed directly to THC. These deaths were not due to single binge overdose, but were nevertheless linked to excessive use of the drug. The *Journal of the Academic of Pediatrics* reported case studies of adolescence succumbing to cerebellar infarctions (strokes) following very heavy marijuana usage. From a physiological perspective, unexpectedly high infusions of THC could cause a drop in blood pressure which may contribute to the stroke. The problem with the statistical evidence for marijuana abuse is that the symptoms of THC and alcohol abuse are rarely seen separately, since the two drugs are usually combined simultaneously. When determining the cause of death, it is just as easy to cite alcohol as it is with marijuana. Nevertheless, when compared to the number of deaths attributed to alcohol overdose (26,000 per year), marijuana statistics can seem much less significant. Yet, alcohol is legal for adults over the age of 21 years, and marijuana is illegal in most states.

Until 2010, the CDC did not record deaths related to anabolic steroid use, but in 2011 it reported three cases of sudden infarction, where steroid use may be involved. From a purely biochemical level, William Taylor identified five pathways through which anabolic steroids can potentially cause heart attacks: (1) atherogenic model, when increased lipoprotein concentrations in the blood form plaque in the arterial walls; (2) thrombus model, resulting from increased clotting factors and platelets; (3) vasospasm, when the vascular nitric oxide system results in a spasm of the arteries; (4) direct myocardial injury model, when the steroids impact the myocardial cells directly; and (5) any combination of the previous four pathways. A Finnish long-range study of 62 powerlifters in 2000 indicated premature death rates four times higher than the general population. Again, these statistics do not amount to causal evidence. Moreover, when compared to the death rates of either marijuana or alcohol, the documented mortality rate of anabolic steroids is extremely low. Yet, for the purposes of cosmetic or performance enhancement, anabolic steroid use is illegal at the federal level.

Nonquantifiable Threats—Risky Lifestyle Choices: Alcohol and Marijuana

When evaluated exclusively on potential health risks, the justification for criminalizing marijuana or anabolic steroids seems to be weaker than the case for criminalizing alcohol. Yet, alcohol is legal for adults and the other two drugs are not. This is because the case for criminalization ultimately rests on factors that go beyond specific health risks. Alcohol, marijuana, and anabolic steroid use are popularly associated with certain lifestyle choices that trigger differing levels of social disruption.

The risks associated with heavy alcohol use begin with a range of routine activities that can become highly dangerous if performed while intoxicated. Driving or operating any motor vehicle and even walking may pose serious risks of injury and death when conducted under the influence of alcohol. Other risks include decisions made as a result of impaired judgment: risky sexual behaviors, including relations with strangers or multiple partners, may result in unintended pregnancies or sexually transmitted diseases. Alcohol also significantly increases the risk of sexual assault and physical violence. Studies from the CDC indicate—two-thirds of all domestic violence cases are alcohol related, and alcohol abuse is the leading cause of child neglect and abuse.

These demonstrable social costs associated with alcohol abuse were among the leading reasons for the prohibition movement in the 1910s and 1920s. The Women's Christian Temperance Union lobbied for public support, using posters with images of women with young children being abandoned at the door of the saloon, while their husbands wasted their money and time inside. They included both statistics and anecdotes of spousal abuse, family neglect, and economic ruin due to uncontrolled alcoholism. The earliest temperance movements of the 1800s sought only to limit alcohol consumption to moderate levels, but after the rapid growth of urbanization following industrialization that priority shifted. The effect of drunkenness on the family, on the neighborhood, and on the moral ethos of an increasingly anonymous urban society convinced activists to seek total prohibition as a necessary safeguard against the threat of alcoholism. By the time of World War I, the demand for moral reform became so strong that 23 of the 48 states passed anti-saloon laws, and by 1919 more than two-thirds of the electorate voted for the Eighteenth Amendment prohibiting the manufacture and sale of alcohol nationwide.

After 13 years, the federal prohibition was overturned. The American public generally accepted the fact that drunkenness lead to social problems, but they did not share a consensus on the need for total prohibition—especially in the urban areas. Immigrant communities were especially unsupportive because mealtime consumption was often interwoven into their cultural traditions of social interaction. In most cases, people drink an alcoholic beverage because they like the taste, or the refreshing effect, or because it is part of their traditions. Even in contemporary times, the CDC reports that only about 28 percent of the population drinks at a level that would put them at risk of intoxication or alcohol dependency. Moderate amounts of alcohol could be consumed for cultural, religious, or culinary purposes with no risk of intoxication at all. By 1933, opponents of prohibition successfully argued that the rights of a majority of responsible drinkers should not be sacrificed by legal prohibitions that are really aimed at the minority of alcohol abusers.

Until the 2000s, there were no similar movements to legalize marijuana. During the 2012 elections, the three states where legalization of marijuana was debated focused mostly on the contrasts between marijuana and alcohol. Advocates for legalizations argued that marijuana was less harmful than alcohol, and since alcohol was legal, then marijuana should also be legal. Opponents argued that the threats were largely social and cultural, and that specific health risks were difficult to quantify. In two of the three elections, voters focused more on the absence of immediate physical risks than they did on the potential cultural threats.

The problem with using statistics to compare the relative risks of alcohol versus marijuana versus anabolic steroids is that the data is not compiled with equal weight. Since alcohol is legal, the actual number of alcohol-related accidents, diseases, and deaths should be higher than the actual numbers of incidents associated with illegal substances. Evidence can be seen with statistics associated with marijuana use, which have been increasing steadily as more states begin to loosen their laws. In 2012, the number of marijuana users reached a 30-year high, with more than three million people added to the ranks between 2009 and 2012. During the same period, the number of emergency rooms visit related to complications involving marijuana also increased significantly, with 375,000 visits in 2011. Likewise, the rate of admissions to drug treatment programs for marijuana addictions increased five times since the 1980s. It is presumed that as more states legalize marijuana the numbers will continue to rise.

From a moral perspective, the primary difference between alcohol and marijuana is the intent of consumption. Statistically, alcohol is consumed most often, by the majority of drinkers, with no deliberate intent to achieve intoxication. Wine or beer is frequently drunk with a meal or used as an ingredient to increase flavor profiles. By contrast, marijuana is consumed almost exclusively with a specific intent to impair judgment. There are no secondary tastes that enhance a meal and the primary object of marijuana use is to achieve some level of intoxication. On a national level, this single-purpose use of marijuana is the primary justification for its continued criminalization.

Numerous longitudinal studies compiled by the National Institute of Drug Abuse indicate that those who smoke pot at young ages are more likely to suffer from poor mental and physical health, endure more relationship problems, cope with more learning difficulties, and generally report less satisfying lives. Heavy marijuana users of all ages are also more likely to suffer from motivational issues leading to higher drop-out rates from school and job loss due to absences, tardiness, and accidents. The possible effects of even minimal marijuana use include damage to short-term memory and intelligence, producing less productive members of society. These social costs are similar to those that follow chronic alcohol abuse, but they are not associated with mild to moderate use of alcohol. The resulting lifestyle of a chronic marijuana user is based on the pursuit of routine inebriation, which removes the individual from the day-to-day stresses of normal social interaction. The same frequency of moderate alcohol use leads to substantially less harmful outcomes than for marijuana use.

Nonquantifiable Threats—Risky Lifestyle Choices: Anabolic Steroids

Popular accounts of personal tragedies associated with anabolic steroid abuse dominate the literature and are far more common than published accounts of safe and moderate consumption. A common theme among the accounts is a sense of uncontrollable addiction. William Taylor was the first to publish scientific studies on the addictive potential for anabolic steroids in the early 1980s, and later researchers published similar findings suggesting a psychological addiction pattern similar to that found among opioids.

Typically, a first time steroid user will observe noticeable increases in muscle mass from low-to-moderate doses when combined with weight training. Personality changes will be noticeable to outside observers, but may not be recognized by the user: a sense of euphoria, increased confidence and self-esteem, sex drive, appetite, and aggressiveness. In addition, users will also experience a mutually reinforcing desire to train more and to use more anabolic steroids. These effects lead to a middle phase of steroid use where the user begins experimenting with various **cycles, stacking,** and **pyramiding** of steroids, which means they take multiple steroids (and other supplements such as creatine, androstenedione, or hGH) at the same time, and alternate different kinds of steroids between cycles. The daily feeding routine of a middle-phase user is dominated by very precise diets, extensive supplements, and intense exercise regimes. The lifestyle change results in further increases in muscle mass and accompanying changes in mood and personality. The user experiences major mood swings, sleep disturbances, and low thresholds of violence and temper. Over time, these personality changes become noticeable to both the user and outside observers. Some disturbing symptoms might include delusions of grandeur followed by bouts of paranoia and episodes of manic excitement followed by bouts of anger. In some cases, psychotic symptoms precede uncontrollable acts of violence and criminal activity.

The psychological dependency of anabolic steroid use results from the mutually reinforcing internal drive mechanism, which stimulates a desire among users to reach higher levels of competition, and therefore use greater amounts of the drug. When the adverse behaviors become noticeable to the user, the attempt to stop using is often overwhelmed by the sense of loss associated with the declining levels of self-confidence and motivation. When the serum steroid level is reduced, users experience an acute hyperadrenergic withdrawal symptom, which often results in depression and suicidal thoughts. As a coping mechanism, users often return to the drug to find relief. In this way, a user becomes psychologically dependent on the drug because they experience an emotional craving for the effects, even if there are no physical signs of addiction. These side effects are difficult to quantify, in so far as they cannot be measured by biochemistry levels or through damage to specific organs. Similarly, it is difficult to objectively measure psychological characteristics such as desire, motivation, and obsession. Nevertheless, William Taylor argues that anabolic steroids may be as psychologically addicting as cocaine, with many of the same reinforcing mechanisms.

It is the lifestyle of the anabolic steroid user that most concerns lawmakers. The popular perception of roid rage derives from the premise that the natural aggressions tied to intense competition unintentionally spills over from the field of performance to personal relationships. The psychological dependency can consume individual priorities and influence routine decision making. This problem is intensified by the clandestine nature of taking illegal steroids, which means that users most often use the drugs outside the supervision of a doctor. Individual users tend to make decisions based on the feedback of their own perceived reactions. The absence of external observers to identify adverse side effects can create a sense of invulnerability as users begin to see themselves as experts. The natural competitive spirit that may have triggered the initial steroid use may be channeled into intense experimentation. The particular combination of stacking and cycling is determined almost exclusively through trial and error. In most gyms that are dedicated to bodybuilding, users rely on steroid gurus, who are amateur athletes who feel so confident about their experience taking steroids that they serve as amateur consultants to other less-experienced users. The gurus may have no medical (or any academic) training at all. The body of data compiled by local gurus is self-fulfilling, insofar as there are few external controls for identifying negative side effects related to mood, aggression, irritability, or priority shifts. The prospective result is a subculture of steroid users, who reinforce, encourage, and promote continued use with few built-in mechanisms that appeal to moderation.

The federal decision in 1990 to include anabolic steroids among the list of Section III controlled substances was the result of an increasing sensitivity to steroids-related disruptions. A series of sensational news stories following the 1988 Olympics, where famous elite athletes (both American and non-American) becoming involved in doping scandals was followed by a series of equally sensational news stories of bodybuilders arrested for violent offenses, including murder. Simultaneously, William Taylor organized a series of lectures to doctors around the country sponsored by Pfizer Laboratories, outlining the epidemic or steroid abuse among professional, amateur, and adolescent athletes. Social pressures increased when the case of Horace Williams made national headlines because he blamed anabolic steroids for pushing him into an apparently random and motiveless murder of a passing transient. Lawmakers did not need to rely exclusively on quantitative measures to base their decisions. Instead, they reacted to the popular perception of the time, which associated anabolic steroids with public disruption.

Like marijuana, anabolic steroids are taken only for the purposes of achieving the desired effects. There is no such thing as steroid use for religious, culinary, or other cultural purposes. As such, even moderate use of anabolic steroids may contribute to a culture of addiction. The scientific community may not have reached consensus on whether steroids can definitively be linked to disruptive behaviors, but at the time of their criminalization, the American public was in agreement. As public perceptions change, so too do the positions of lawmakers and policy makers. The question of whether the use of anabolic steroids for nontherapeutic purposes, which constitutes a threat to anyone outside the individual user, continues to be debated.

ARGUMENTS FOR AND AGAINST LEGALITY OF ANABOLIC STEROIDS FOR NONTHERAPEUTIC USES

Nationwide discussions of whether anabolic steroids should continue to be criminalized emerged just around the same time as national debates arose concerning the legalization of marijuana for recreational use. Though the two drugs are completely unrelated in their biochemical classification, they share a common tie, insofar as their criminalization is based on risks that are not always easily quantifiable—either due to the presence of other variables in long-term health risks (which may not be perfectly understood) or as a result of lifestyle choices that are potentially disruptive to the public good.

As the sense of what constitutes public good began to change in the 2000s, more emphasis was placed on physical individual health than on the moral health of the society. As such, the justifications for continued criminalization faced increasing challenges. The question at issue is whether the particular social risks that would follow the legalization of anabolic steroids rise to a level that requires specific legal prohibition (like cocaine), or whether they should be included among those risks that each individual can decide for themselves (like alcohol).

For Legalization

In an article titled "Why Steroids Should Be Legal" written for the website *www.anabolic-steroids.info*, David Steen wrote, "Testosterone and related compounds are neither toxic nor addictive. . . . The use of anabolic steroids can certainly cause side-effects, just as the use of most other medicaments. But there is no serious medical study proving the relation between use of anabolic steroids and serious disease." These two presumptions form the beginning basis for most arguments advocating for legalization: (1) the quantifiable health risks are minimal and (2) there are other drugs that are legally available, which have worse side effects. David Steen wrote for a popular pro-steroid website, but the key elements may be found in almost any publication advocating legalization. Other specific conclusions may vary from individual to individual, but most arise from these two presuppositions.

In a 1994 article written for the *Loyola of Los Angeles Entertainment Law Journal*, John Burge provided a legal justification for reforming existing drug laws related to anabolic steroids. He adds to the standard argument an observation that American entertainment culture provides very strong incentives for athletic victory, including wealth, fame, and respect. Elite athletes can earn multimillion dollar salaries, including near-equivalent sums in endorsements, and are followed by millions of adoring fans. In such an environment, the legal prohibitions against drugs that have been shown to be effective in improving performance stand little chance of influencing individual decision making. As a result, the illicit use of anabolic steroids is virtually uncontrollable, with most elite athletes as well as a strong percentage of amateur athletes and noncompeting individuals using them.

Since Burge also assumed there were no quantifiable health risks to individuals or to others, he concluded that the incentives for using steroids far outweigh the liabilities, thereby creating a massive underground market to meet the demand. The most significant social cost of continued criminalization is that it creates a subculture that removes the athlete from the responsible oversight of doctors (in administering the drug) and the FDA (in the controlled manufacture and supply of the drug). Burge's recommended solution was to legalize anabolic steroids for ergogenic and cosmetic use as long as it was administered under strict physician supervision (to account for any potential health risks that might arise in each individual.)

In 2008, an international panel of experts came together in a debate covered by the National Public Radio to discuss the formal proposition that anabolic steroids should be accepted in competitive sports. The question of legalization was incidental, but reflected the same core question about whether the risks of the drugs were significant enough to warrant prohibition (either by private sports associations or by civil government). A professor of pediatrics and bioethics at the University of Wisconsin, Norman Frost, argued, "Anabolic steroids do have undesirable side effects: acne, baldness, voice changes . . . infertility. But sport itself is far more dangerous, and we don't prohibit it." If we allow individuals to plunge down a hillside at nearly 100 miles an hour on skis or a luge sled, then athletes should be able to make decisions as to whether they want to accept the potential health risks of anabolic steroids.

Underlying each of these arguments is a presupposition that the only relevant health risks are those that are quantifiably linked in a causal relationship between anabolic steroids and serious disease. The threat of a lifestyle of risky behaviors does not enter into the calculus. Similarly, the threat of roid rage is presumed to be more mythical than scientific. In part, the support for legalization reflects deeper sentiments that are hostile to the moral presumptions that originally underlay criminalization. During the same 2008 debate, the senior editor of *Reason* magazine, Radley Balko explained, "So what is this debate really all about? I'd suggest it's about paternalism, and it's about control. We have a full-blown moral panic on our hands here, and it's over a set of substances that, for whatever reason, has attracted the ire of the people who have made it their job to tell us what is and isn't good for us." Balko's argument assumes that the only compelling reason for criminalization is its possible moral effect on the individual and society. Since Balko does not consider those reasons to be pertinent in a modern, pluralistic society, he naturally finds no compelling reason to continue criminalization.

Balko's rejection of moral criteria for evaluating social risk was echoed by Julian Savulescu, a professor of practical ethics at the University of Oxford. He compared the risks of ergogenic drugs with alcohol, and suggested, "To say that we should reduce drugs in sport or eliminate them because they increase performance, is simply like saying that we should eliminate alcohol from parties because it increases sociability." In previous eras, however, this is precisely what people said about alcohol. The risky behaviors that accompany the impaired judgment associated with alcohol use were the main reason why some college campuses are dry and why the WCTU lobbied for criminalization in the 1910s. In a similar way, those arguing against legalization of steroids often do so because they are concerned about the moral impact on individual and society. If, as Savulescu implies, the public presumptions of moral risk have changed since the 1920s, then those arguments could be less compelling.

For Criminalization

The larger majority of policy makers are still committed to maintaining existing criminal prohibitions for anabolic steroid use. Most observers, whether they support or oppose legalization, freely acknowledge the fact that anabolic steroids will significantly enhance athletic performance and lead to increased endurance, muscle growth, and faster healing times. The critical difference is that the advocates for continued criminalization believe much more strongly that anabolic steroids pose health risks, both immediate and long term. The absence of clinical evidence to positively demonstrate the causal relationship between steroids and serious disease is misleading. Arguments of negation cannot be used to assert positive conclusions. The correlative studies linking the drugs to a host of adverse conditions are both consistent and significant, which means that there must be a causal connection somewhere. Just as there are no absolute conclusions that tie anabolic steroids to cardiac infarctions, liver disease, or certain cancers, so too there are no definitive clinical studies that absolutely rule out the connection. The majority of arguments in support of continued criminalization presuppose such physical risks.

In addition, though, the threshold for legal prohibition requires not only a presumption of personal health risks, but it must also include some probable threat of public disruption. Cigarette smoke and deep-fried fast foods lead to demonstrable health risks if consumed on a regular basis, but there is little evidence to suggest that those risks extend to anyone other than the individual. Only when the risk of second-hand cigarette smoke became popularly associated with serious respiration disorders were users frequently prohibited from smoking in public spaces where the ventilation was confined. In the case of anabolic steroids, the advocates for continued criminalization believe strongly that ergogenic use significantly increases the risks of aggressive behaviors, violent outbursts, and psychological addiction that can potentially result both in criminal activity necessary to support the habit and increased suicide risks among those trying to quit.

During the Senate Hearings that preceded the Steroid Trafficking Act of 1990, which was the legal basis for classifying anabolic steroids as a Schedule III controlled substance, Senator Joseph Biden (D-DE) listed four reasons for criminalizing steroid use for nontherapeutic purposes. First, he argued that it "threatens the mental and physical welfare" of those most likely to be in healthy condition. Second, Biden believed anabolic steroids would serve as a gateway drug. As he explained, "If young people accept the idea that using steroids to build their body is okay, they may be all the more likely to try other drugs to alter their minds, as well as their bodies." Third, he warned that "using drugs to improve athletic performance undermines our most basic notions of honesty, discipline and hard work as a means for achieving." And fourth, protecting the health and well-being of elite athletes was critical, "Because," as Biden explained, "they are role models for all people, not just athletes, and young people." These four justifications remain the core reasons for continued criminalization of anabolic steroids.

Of the four reasons listed, the first two reiterate the basic conviction that anabolic steroids are not only harmful to individuals, but to others as well. The latter two reasons reflect less quantifiable justifications related to risky lifestyle choices and inappropriate role modeling. As the arguments in favor of legalizations imply, perhaps the most influential arguments are those related to public morality. Steroids promote a culture that emphasizes winning over all other priorities, including physical health and moral character (particularly honesty, perseverance, and humility). Whether the competitive spirit emerges through formal athletic events or through informal social interactions, the emphasis on material measures of success and happiness can have a detrimental impact on social values. Honest self-assessment, which may include recognizing personal weaknesses, inevitably plays a secondary consideration behind public pressures for social conformity.

During the 2008 forum debating whether anabolic steroids should be allowed in sports, the chairman of the World Anti-Doping Agency, Richard Pound, argued that ergogenic drugs contributed to social pressures that were fundamentally destructive both to the spirit of sport and to principles upon which civil society relied. He explained, "The use of performance-enhancing drugs is not accidental; it is planned and deliberate with the sole objective of getting an unfair advantage. I don't want my kids, or your kids, or anybody's kids to have to turn themselves into chemical stockpiles just because there are cheaters out there who don't care what they promised when they started to participate. I don't want my kids in the hands of a coach who would encourage or allow the use of drugs among his or her athletes." The risk to physical health is critical to Pound's conviction, but it is not the only concern. He suggests that even if steroids were not a health risk, they would still be culturally detrimental because those who take them do so with deliberate intentions to undermine the rules. Such priorities place their chances of winning at a higher level than honesty, integrity, or individual moral restraint.

Moral Order and Practical Liberty in Civil Society

In a civil society, lawmakers are often faced with two competing priorities when they codify criminal law. On the one hand, the society needs to protect against disruptions that undermine the individual rights of others. On the other hand, in the pursuit of that protection, society may unfairly limit the individual right to pursue their own happiness in a manner they best deem fitting. The tension is most apparent for questions dealing with public morality and the dangers of individual lifestyle choices. In a civil society, individuals are presumed free to make any choice that does not create a public disruption. Lawmakers must demonstrate genuine harm to justify legal prohibition against an individual's freedom to make their own lifestyle choices.

According to those who support continued criminalization of anabolic steroids, the prospective threat is measurable in correlative terms (increased disease rates among users), but the direct causal connections is not always quantifiable. According to those who support legalization, if the risks to the greater society are not quantified by specific causal evidence, then lawmakers should err on the side of caution and leave the decisions for assuming (or avoiding) potential risks to the individual user.

LEGALIZATION OF CIGARETTES?

Public debates occurred over the legalization (and criminalization) of alcohol in the 1910s/1920s and of marijuana in the 2010s. Future debates may arise over the criminalization of cigarettes. A 2006 national opinion poll indicated that 45 percent of Americans said they would be willing to criminalize cigarettes in the next 5 or 10 years. Among those who responded, the 18–29-year-olds reported the highest support for criminalization (57%), while those aged 50–64 years reported the lowest amount of support (40%). In 2012, Oregon lawmaker Mitch Greenlick made such a proposal in this own state (it was defeated). The eventual outcome of such debates will depend largely on whether the public threat is viewed exclusively as a risk to physical health or more broadly as a threat to existing cultural priorities.

FEDERAL ISSUES

Another aspect of the criminalization debate that is rarely discussed is the role of federalism in a lawmaker's decisions to legalize and criminalize a drug. Federalism means that independent governing bodies coexist at both the individual state and the federal levels. In most cases that do not involve the due process of law, there is no automatic priority between federal and state laws. The Tenth Amendment guarantees that all powers that are not expressly delegated to the federal government are reserved for the state government. For more than century, this meant that those laws related to criminal prosecution were handled at the state level. The federal government did not get involved in local crimes because there were always local officials that were geographically closer and who had a closer, more personal perspective on the crime.

Issues of federalism became most pronounced during the mid-1850s, as lawmakers debated whether state (or the federal) government most held the right to determine if slavery was compatible for established civil rights. The South argued that the states alone made such determinations, while the North argued that the federal government was the ultimate defender of certain core rights (including life and liberty). The Fourteenth Amendment was passed following the southern defeat during the Civil War, and it explicitly gave the federal government the jurisdiction (and obligation) to provide a minimum level of rights for all Americans, regardless of what state they resided in. The primary intent was originally to protect the rights of the newly freed slaves, but over time, the Fourteenth Amendment has been used to guarantee certain rights among all defendants in criminal cases regardless of whether it is handled at the state or federal level. Since criminal laws all involve due process, the federal government has become the dominant authority in matters related to criminal procedures.

Local and state officials are still the primary enforcers of the law, and their enforcement deals mostly with local and state ordinances. Nevertheless, the federal government remains the last source of appeal. This can create a dilemma of jurisdiction. For example, in 1919, the federal constitution was amended to prohibit the manufacture and sale of alcohol for recreational use. For just under half the country, the law had little direct bearing because the citizens in 23 of the 48 states had already passed similar laws at the state level. As a practical matter, prohibition suffered major problems of enforcement because for those states, where alcohol was not already prohibited, the primary law enforcement officer was the federal prohibition agent. Prior to 1920, there were barely a handful of federal agents in any agency. During the height of prohibition, the number of agents increased significantly, but it was never more than the number of policemen in New York City—and the federal agents were responsible for patrolling the entire country. The practical decision to enforce a criminal ordinance must be shared at both the federal and state levels for a given law to be effective.

On the other side of the issue, a federal government repeal of a federal law does not necessarily impact state laws. When the Eighteenth Amendment was repealed by the Twenty-First Amendment in 1933, it did not necessarily mean that alcohol was legal in all states. Mississippi did not end prohibition until 1966. There are many counties, including the famous

Bourbon County in Kentucky (for which Kentucky Bourbon is named), which continue to prohibit the sale of alcohol to the present day. This means that any state that currently prohibits the sale of anabolic steroids for nontherapeutic uses would continue to prohibit that activity, even if the drug was removed from the federal list of controlled substances.

The practical problem of enforcement is more relevant when a state chooses to decriminalize a substance that is listed among the controlled substances at the federal level. In 1996, California became the first state to legalize marijuana for medical use. Since marijuana is listed as a Schedule I controlled substance, the federal government did not recognize therapeutic uses for the drug. This created a contradiction between state and federal enforcement officers. At the federal level, the manufacture and distribution of marijuana remained a federal offense. Over the course of the next 15 years, nearly 20 states followed California's example, and the open conflict between federal and state jurisdiction widened. In 2009, President Barack Obama sent a memo to federal prosecutors recommending that they not prosecute marijuana offences in states that have legalized the drug for medical use. He reiterated the recommendation again in 2013. The memo was an executive decision, however, and other presidential administrations may choose to rescind the practice. In such cases, it would be up to the courts to decide who held ultimate jurisdiction.

These jurisdictional issues are relevant to anabolic steroids because the effort to decriminalize the drug could come from either state or federal levels. If California chose to legalize anabolic steroids for recreational use, then the federal government would have to decide whether it would prosecute offenders at the federal level. At the same time, legalization at the federal level does not mean that local and private associations must allow the same behaviors. That means that a legal steroid may still be prohibited in either professional or amateur sports.

CONCLUSION

Anabolic steroids have been illegal without a prescription since the 1980s, and were criminalized for nontherapeutic use since 1990. Yet, the prevalence of anabolic steroids does not seem to be declining in the realm of professional and amateur sports. The tools for detection have improved significantly, but the strategies for evasion seem to be equally innovative. One of the more common arguments for legalization is that the laws do not have a noticeable impact on either the demand or the supply of the drugs. Why then should they continue to be outlawed?

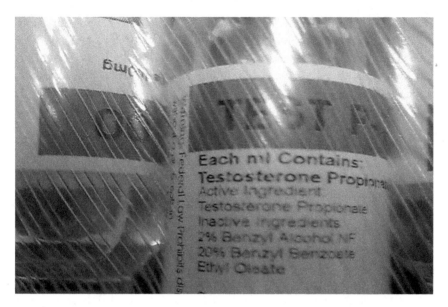

The Drug Enforcement Agency confiscated vials of anabolic steroids during Operation Raw Deal in 2007. (Drug Enforcement Agency)

For the most part, the answer is that the public generally believes that open legalization would cause more harm to society than continued criminalization. Of specific concern is the impact of what would be viewed as an official government endorsement of anabolic steroids for nontherapeutic use. If the government makes a drug legal, then it is saying that the risks associated with the drug are not significant enough to warrant intervention. Popular use would increase significantly—perhaps, especially among youth who have not yet developed a sense of delayed gratification and who would face little reason to resist the temptation. In effect, the criminalization of anabolic steroids is a reflection of the public concern for the impact on public morality.

From a philosophical perspective, there is a legitimate question of whether a civil society can ever truly fix a social problem through legislation alone. Experts in the fields of biochemistry, medicine, sociology, and psychology could theoretically devise a perfect society designed to protect all people, to limit all risks, and ensure the greatest well-being for the largest number of people. Unfortunately, such laws are only effective if the general public agrees to adhere to them. Crime will exist as long as an individual chooses to place their decisions at a higher priority than society's guidelines. To completely eliminate crime, society would have to completely eliminate individual free will—and that violates the spirit of the civil society.

Therein lay the central controversy to the question of legalized steroids: should society reduce the rights and opportunities of all people in order to limit the potential of abusive behaviors exhibited by a few? If the threat posed by those few is deemed to be great enough, the answer is yes. If not, the answer is no. Defining what constitutes a threat to the public order becomes much more complicated when we include nonquantifiable elements, such as long-term risks and self-destructive lifestyle choices. The more heavily the criminalization of anabolic steroids relies on threats to public morality, the greater the opening for critics to argue that their individual rights are being unnecessarily hindered. At the same time, the more often that the movement for legalization is limited exclusively to the absence of causal evidence, the greater the opportunity for opponents to charge selfish indifference to explain the decline of public morality.

The question of legality also poses a very difficult dilemma for private sports associations and other entities, who periodically review their anti-doping policies. On the one hand, the sports association's policies reflect a common consensus with the civil government's decision to legally prohibit the drugs. The history of the anti-doping initiatives reveals a slow process of an emerging consensus over the health risks of ergogenic drugs. The sports community acts on the belief that unfettered access to anabolic steroids is fundamentally harmful to the athlete. On the other, the vast majority of public debates over anabolic steroids occur within the arena of sports media. Every time a new headline of a sports hero caught using steroids comes up, the fans and commentators alike debate the wisdom of potential rule changes among sports associations to allow ergogenic drugs. As a practical matter, no real change could occur until and unless the question of criminality changes first. Yet, the pressure for changing civil laws may not arise unless the sports community first changes its position, which presupposes significant health risks to the athletes and cultural risks to the sport itself. In terms of timing, the prospect for changing the direction of existing laws prohibiting the nontherapeutic use of anabolic steroids is relatively low.

The next chapter discusses some of the issues involved with sports association decisions to regulate the use of ergogenic supplements among their members. Discussions will include specific issues related to amateur and professional anti-doping policies, as well as brief summaries of some of the more famous athletes involved in steroid scandals.

CHAPTER 6

Anti-Doping within Organizations

In his book, *Anabolic Steroids in Sports and Exercise*, Charles Yesalis explained that there "were a number of ironies" associated with sports associations being asked to regulate their own anti-doping programs. He argued that anabolic steroids were originally invented by scientists to satisfy a growing demand from the sports community for new chemicals to make athletes stronger, faster, and more enduring. Yet, this same sports community is also being asked to develop ways to stop drug use among athletes. Yesalis sympathized with athletes told by officials to resist anabolic steroids, but are also told by their coaches and trainers that only the highest levels of performance will lead to national success. Moreover, they were also bombarded with streams of commercials and images that promise new pills to solve almost any problem. The pressures are not compatible with each other—one set seeks to push athletes beyond all limits and the other seeks to establish unbreakable barriers. Yesalis doubted that a meaningful anti-doping program could work without somehow aligning these forces toward the same goal.

As an academic researcher, Yesalis first began publishing studies on the effect of steroids on athletes in the 1970s. On several occasions in the late 1980s, he served as an expert witness on the subject before lawmakers, who were considering the legal status of performance-enhancing steroids. Sometimes referred to as an anti-doping crusader, Yesalis was outspoken in his opposition to the forces that seem to encourage ergogenic drug use in sports. He explained, "Not only did the medical community develop these drugs, but it played a role early on in 'selling' this potential fountain of youth." On the global stage, physicians, government scientists, and certain sports officials in communist nations were at the forefront of developing new ergogenic drugs to undermine official rules at international sporting events. At home in the United States, physicians and coaching staffs at the professional, collegiate, and even some high school teams began experimenting and supplying ergogenic drugs to improve their team's performances. Yesalis argued, "It was a number of sport federations that for decades covered up this problem, conveniently looked the other way, or instituted drug-testing programs that were designed to fail. . . . It was (and is) our society that emphasizes and rewards speed, strength, size, aggression, and winning."

Yesalis was not pointing the finger at any particular individual official in the anti-doping community. Instead, he was emphasizing the fact that the sports industry seems to provide more incentives than disincentives for athletes to use ergogenic drugs. Any effective effort to limit or end doping in sports requires genuine changes in cultural priorities. Yesalis supported the federal government's reclassification of anabolic steroids as a Schedule III controlled substance when used for the purposes of performance enhancement because he believed the risk to public health is very high. At the same time, he also argued that government prohibition was not sufficient to curb individual use because law enforcement officials necessarily concentrate their efforts on the suppliers (drug dealers) and not on the users. The risk of fines or jail time for inappropriately using anabolic steroids is fairly low. Therefore, the sectors of society that, potentially, have the greatest effect in deterring ergogenic drug use are those who most often interact with the athletes: the professional and amateur sports associations, the high school coaches, and even the sports media. Unless these associations make a sincere effort to create a culture within the athletic community that encourages chemical-free competition, then the threat of criminal consequences will have little impact.

The difficulty facing most sports associations is that they must match their sincere anti-doping policies against strong public pressures for more exciting sports events. The potential for organizing professional and amateur venues is largely dependent on the promise of money raised through public interest. The higher the interest, the greater the resources available for sports associations to hire officials, procure facilities, attract new players, and retain existing players. Ergogenic drugs increase the performance of most athletes, leading to more sensational competition, which improves the financial success of sports associations. Yet, this kind of success also leads to increasing risks to the physical, psychological, and moral well-being of their players. It is out of a genuine desire to protect the health of their players that sports associations have cooperated with international anti-doping efforts, but as Yesalis suggests, the efforts have not always been eagerly embraced. Considerable debate remains over whether the anti-doping policies are implemented with a sincere attempt to curb drug use or whether they are intended to encourage athletes to be more effective at hiding their use.

THE ROLE OF ASSOCIATIONS IN IDENTIFYING CULTURAL PRIORITIES

Lawmakers demonstrated a commitment to sanctioning anabolic steroid use for performance enhancement, but there is significant discussion over whether American society shares that same commitment. In part, the question stems from the universal application of the law, which only distinguishes between medical and nonmedical purposes and not between the kinds of nontherapeutic uses. Some of the questions raised include: if the livelihood of professional athletes rests on their ability to sustain strong performance over the course of their career, should exceptions be made to distinguish them from other amateur athletes? Should distinctions be made between collegiate athletes who demonstrate potential for a professional career and high school-level athletes who may only be pursuing an extracurricular activity?

Public discussions of such questions usually focus on fairness and the inevitable impact on competition between players that do not use ergogenic drugs. There are, however, other considerations outside the competition. For example, if soldiers or law enforcement officers already place their lives at risk for the sake of protecting the peace of the community, then should exceptions be made to allow them every advantage afforded by ergogenic drugs? These questions may be discussed within the confines of each group's representative associations (professional sports, collegiate sports, police associations, military hierarchies), but the ultimate question of legality remains in the hands of lawmakers. Any meaningful exceptions would require specific legal changes.

Other kinds of associations may discuss the nontherapeutic use of steroids without requiring changes to the classification of anabolic steroids as a controlled substance. For example, the use of steroids on animals is mostly determined by industrial associations. For competitive racing, the primary questions focus on the potential for fraud related to gambling, as well as the potential cruelty to animals. Outside the competition, questions deal mostly with food safety. For example, should agricultural specialists use performance-enhancing hormones on their animals to produce higher yields of milk, meat, or hair/fur? What effect do specialized growth hormones injected in animals have on the humans that eat them? These questions are usually discussed within the related agricultural associations, and their decisions may or may not involve government regulation or legislative action.

Lawmakers chose to treat all anabolic steroids for performance enhancement in the same way as a Schedule III controlled substance, because a single classification sends a strong message of disapproval for the nontherapeutic use of such drugs. Yet, other cultural incentives available for elite-level athletes who demonstrate exceptional performance create conflicting messages. Associations of professional and amateur athletes, as well as other civic and industrial groups, can play a significant role in managing the level of cultural dissonance by reinforcing priorities that either support or contradict the spirit of the existing laws. If the associations generally support the spirit of the laws that criminalize nontherapeutic use of anabolic steroids, then the cultural trend will be toward a gradual reduction of ergogenic drug use. If the associations generally undermine the spirit of the laws, then our democratic society will likely see a future change in the laws. In either case, sports and other associations play a significant role in defining the public will.

THE IDEOLOGY BEHIND ANTI-DOPING POLICIES

The international anti-doping movement arose first among international sports associations during the 1920s, though enforcement was impossible since no tests had yet been invented to detect the ergogenic drugs. Athletes were held by their honor to refrain from using chemicals to enhance their performance. As such, any accusations of violations often involved more than merely breaking the rules; the athletes' honor was at question, as was the honor of their coaches, trainers, and even their home country. As long as there were no tests that could provide absolute proof one way or another, then the question of doping was largely relegated to rumors. This background to the first anti-doping policies is important because it demonstrates the complex balancing act that enforcers must try to maintain.

Anti-Doping Diplomacy

During the 1960s, several famous incidents—including the death of two cyclists, Knud Jensen (1960) and Tom Simpson (1967)—served to pressure the International Olympic Committee (IOC) to develop more systematic testing procedures for existing anti-doping rules. Most other national and international sports associations tended to follow the IOC lead. Nevertheless, the process was slow to be implemented, and it was almost a decade before athletes faced any real threat of detection. During the implementation phase, the IOC launched an education campaign that emphasized the need to protect athletes from drugs that could pose serious health risks, and the need to protect the integrity of the games by insuring each performance represented the best human potential (and not the best chemistry). Player safety and an equal playing field were the standard justifications for the increasing number of policies and procedures necessary to implement an effective anti-doping program. These two justifications were relatively safe to assert and difficult to oppose.

Throughout the period of transition, before systematic drug testing became fully implemented, there remained some strong (if less vocal) voices of opposition. Most criticism was indirect because few athletes, or coaches, or national sports associations wanted to be on record as opposing player safety or equal playing fields. Instead, the opposition was veiled behind other issues that were legitimate concerns that anyone could raise. For example, coaches and trainers initially feared the threat of unintended violations—how were athletes around the world going to be properly informed about the proscriptions and expectations of the testing procedures? Another issue related to privacy—urine tests required officials to actually watch the urine stream as it filled the container to make sure it came directly from the tested athlete and not from some other source. Coaches, trainers, and athletes could raise legitimate concerns, since the testing could be embarrassing. Also, since the early tests were expensive, there were fears that the athletes of some countries would be unfairly targeted for testing, while others were ignored. Similarly, some athletes worried that the tests were not accurate and may lead to false positives, or might detect substances that were legal and identify them as contraband. Some drugs that are legally used for therapeutic purposes to treat non-sports-related ailments may trigger a bad drug test. These and other issues forced the IOC to not only continually modify their procedures for the sake of equity, but also to repeat their justifications that the benefits of the new anti-doping rules outweighed the inconveniences of drug testing—and far outweighed the consequence that would follow if there were no tests at all.

Part of the reason for tensions related to the implementation of anti-doping programs is that by their very nature they seem to challenge the integrity of the athlete, the coach/training staff, and the national sports associations. In the 1930s, an athlete's word was all that was needed (and indeed, it was all that was possible to extract) to ensure safe and equitable playing field. By the 1980s, the athlete had to add samples of hair, urine, and/or blood to their personal declarations. Any positive test meant that at some point in the local sports community—either the athlete, or the trainer, or coach, or the even the national association—someone was complicit in lying to the officials and attempting to cheat. In order to maintain some sense of objectivity, and to avoid the conflict of exchanges where honor and reputation was at stake, the IOC followed a policy of restraint with regard to its doping allegations; unless there was specific factual evidence to support the claim, the IOC did not accuse any individual or country of abuse nor did it publicly challenge a country's stated commitment to anti-doping programs.

Anti-Doping Politics

The increasing numbers of positive tests attest to the fact that some athletes did violate their pledges, they did lie to officials, and they did cheat. Details of other scandals (such as the Festina incident during the 1998 Tour de France) also showed that coaches and trainers were sometimes directly involved in planning and organizing the doping. In some cases, the collusion extended even to the national level. After the Soviet Union collapsed in the 1990s, former East German officials were tried for their part in the systematic doping of their athletes in an attempt to evade IOC detection methods. These scandals were newsworthy because the conspirators were caught, but there was no surprise that such conspiracies existed. Rumors of national collusion were voiced as early as the 1936 Berlin Olympics, when future IOC President Avery Brundage voiced his skepticism that some of the German women athletes were actually men (in fact, German high jumper Dora Ratgen was discovered after the war to be male—Hermann Ratgen—and had been forced by Nazi officials to hide his genitals in order to compete as a woman). In the 1950s, numerous coaches suspected that the East German Weightlifting team was taking some form of testosterone (which the U.S. Team physician John Ziegler later affirmed). In the 1990s, the suspicion was shifted to Chinese and North Korean athletes. The rumors and allegations of some degree of national conspiracy have become common at all international events.

The official IOC position was to avoid commenting on such rumors without specific factual evidence, but there were little doubt that some countries and some trainers, or coaches, or athletes were more likely than others to conspire to evade anti-doping procedures. Starting with the Hitler's hosting of the 1936 Berlin Olympics, certain international competitions have become forums for national propaganda campaigns. This became extremely common during the Cold War, when the Communist Bloc countries attempted to use the Olympic successes of their athletes as a political statement to somehow justify the superiority of their economic systems. The duplicitous nature of a totalitarian regime often means that the national spokespersons will claim total compliance with any and all anti-doping policies, and yet, at the same time, deliberately seek methods for undermining them—in other words, they lie. Throughout the early 1990s, the coaches of the suddenly victorious Chinese swim team repeatedly claimed that their wins were due to sophisticated training programs and the natural superiority of their athletes and coaches, and that they absolutely forbade any use of steroids or other banned drugs. Yet, in 1994, a surprise drug test revealed that 11 of their top swimmers had been using DHT. Very shortly thereafter, a routine airport security check on an athlete of the same team led to numerous vials of hGH.

In such situations, when the nation's honor is at stake, the international anti-doping community must resist the temptation to make accusations of national conspiracy lest they find themselves embroiled in countercharges of partiality or national favoritism. The tensions involved with elite-level competition are rarely limited to simple questions of compliance. After the 2012 Olympics, when Jamaican sprinters Usain Bolt and Yohan Blake came in first and second with record-breaking times, suspicion emerged that the Jamaican anti-doping agency (JADCO) had failed to adequately test its athletes. The suspicions arose, in part, because the 10-second 100-meter barrier had remained unbroken for 60 years until Jim Hines raced it in 9.95 seconds in 1968. One athlete repeated the feat in 1977 and three more did so in the early 1980s. After 1988, the barrier was broken 80 times, and 25 percent of those athletes were later found to have used steroids or some other ergogenic drug. During the Olympic finals in 2012, seven of the eight sprinters broke the 10-second barrier. In 2013, five Jamaican runners tested positive, including Bolt's teammate Asafa Powell and female sprinter Sherone Simpson. After the news, the former executive director of JADCO, Renee Anne Shirley, released a statement claiming that there were flaws in her organization's testing procedures and that the Jamaican sports association often met her suggestions for correction with open hostility. For their part, the Jamaican Olympic Committee responded immediately with allegations that Shirley and others were trying to discredit their organization. Though Usain Bolt failed no tests, public opinion polls following the incident indicated just under 50 percent suspect some organized drug use. Yet, without specific evidence, all such suspicions remain rumors and the official IOC policy is to ignore them until proven otherwise. The World Anti-Doping Agency responded with a brief message saying that they hoped a full investigation would follow, but made no other accusations.

Coercion—The Other Unspoken Justification

For these reasons, the official and most quoted justifications for international anti-doping policies are limited to ensuring athlete safety and maintaining equal playing field. Beyond these two, however, the other justifications that most trainers/coaches recognize, even if they do not always find expression in official documentation, is the risk of athletes being drugged without their free and voluntary consent. In nondemocratic countries, there is always some suspicion that the government may use various forms of explicit or implicit coercion to compel their athletes to victory.

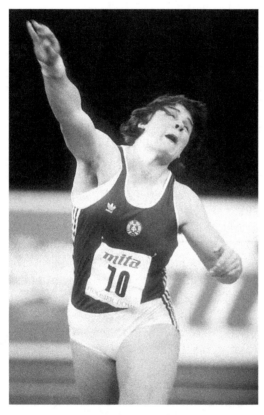

Olympic champion shot-putter Heidi Krieger of East Germany competes during the Women's shot-put event at the 1987 World Indoor Athletics Championships, held in the Hoosier Dome in Indianapolis in early March 1987. Krieger, one of many athletes to participate in the covert but systemic East German doping program, later undertook a sex change operation due the masculinization caused by years of steroid abuse at the insistence of coaches. (Tony Duffy/Getty Images)

In 2000, 10 years after the collapse of the Soviet Union and German reunification, Manfred Ewald and Manfred Höeppner were tried and convicted of causing "intentional bodily harm of athletes, including minors." Ewald served as sports minister for East Germany from 1961 to 1988, and Höeppner served as his chief medical director. Together, they designed a government-sponsored program to provide anabolic steroids and other ergogenic drugs to an estimated 10,000 athletes during their tenures. Many of the athletes were under the age of 16 and were told to take vitamins and supplements, which included various forms of testosterone. Evidence presented at their trial included 142 cases of cancer, ovarian cysts, liver dysfunction, and birth defects in their children. One athlete, Heidi Krieger, said that her steroid use resulted in so many secondary male characteristics that she eventually chose to undergo a sex reassignment surgery to complete the process that had begun during her Olympic training. Other cases of emotional and psychological disorders were included as evidence. Former swimming champion, Martina Gottschalk, testified, "I can't forget what was done to me. . . . Three times a day we had to swallow little blue pills with sweetened tea. We were told it was vitamins, but we were doped against our will." She said she still suffered from pains in her abdomen, dysfunction with her gall bladder, and she attributed her son's birth defect to the steroid use. More than 500 people—coaches, trainers, and doctors—were involved in the program and were being investigated by German authorities.

The East German doping program was exposed largely because the country collapsed and the communist regime was willingly discredited by the new unified German republic. Yet, there are other totalitarian governments in the world that do not voluntarily disclose the details of their training programs. There are numerous unconfirmed rumors of similar style programs, particularly in China and North Korea. No explicit evidence has been uncovered, and so the international community resists open accusations and the IOC operates on the assumption that the national anti-doping policies are being fully enforced.

Voluntary Coercion?

While the totalitarian governments face the greatest suspicion of national conspiracies, they are not alone. In 2008, the German Olympic Sports Confederation and its Federal Institute of Sport Science commissioned a report to look into the sports program of West Germany between the 1950s and the 1990s. The 800-page report revealed consistent use of amphetamines during the World Cup soccer matches and long-term

conspiracies between politicians, doctors, and other officials in the nation's Olympic program. Evidence indicated that the chief physician for
the West Germany Olympic Teams routinely pursued less public strategies
for removing anabolic steroids from the IOCs list of banned drugs. Suspicions of West German doping conspiracy received international attention
in 1987 after heptathlete Birgit Dressel died at the age of 26 from multiple
organ failures. Though her death was attributed to unknown causes, her
autopsy revealed more than 100 different medicines in her system.

Unlike her eastern sister, West Germany was a democratic republic,
which means athletes were not compelled to participate. Yet, the question of
coercion remains strong. As one West German sports official quoted by the
2008 report explained, "Coaches always told me that, if you don't take anything, you will not become something. Anyone who became something was
taking [steroids]." This kind of pressure may not involve threats of physical
or economic reprisal, but it nevertheless limits the options of the athlete to
make their own decisions about their training regimen. The coaches, trainers, and officials created an environment which assumed that steroid-based
enhancement was necessary for successful competition, and therefore any
unwillingness to participate would be seen as a lack of commitment.

In both the West and East German sports programs, athletes were placed
in a position where they were forced to choose between their health and the
rewards associated with elite competition. Critics who read the 2008 report argued that it did not matter whether the official organization framed
the decision to use steroids as an external mandate or a personal decision.
In both instances, the athlete faced a coercive environment. It was this kind
of social pressure that was most frequently alluded to during the Congressional hearings of the late 1980s, which debated whether or not to include
anabolic steroids among the list of controlled substances in the United
States. When high school or college youths are thrust into an environment
where their coaches, trainers, or other adult mentors promote the use of
steroids as a necessary part of a competition, then there is some argument
that the youth is being effectively coerced into drug use. Their age and lack
of experience prevents them from making informed decisions. The criminalization of anabolic steroids for performance enhancement helped to
limit the public endorsements of the drug, but prohibitions against private
or personal recommendations from mentors are not enforceable.

Moral Concerns—The Difficult Justification

Yesalis argued that the only effective anti-doping program is to change
public attitudes. He warned that "if we cannot control our competitive and

narcissistic natures, we then must resign ourselves to anabolic steroid use, even among our children." Individual player safety and equality on the playing field are the first justifications for anti-doping policies, but Yesalis would argue that they are symptoms of a deeper challenge to public morality. Athletes who use drugs to enhance their performance are willingly breaking the rules of competition and placing their health and welfare at risk, all for the sake of victory. This approach undermines the spirit of personal development and encourages a more utilitarian priority where the end justifies the means.

The difficulty with making moral arguments is that they presume common standards of natural law. During the 1800s, in the age of Pierre de Coubertin, few questioned the moral value of sportsmanship as a path to character development. The distinction between amateur and professional athletes was based on a premise that those who refused pay for their sport (the amateurs) recognized the intrinsic value of competition as a personal challenge. Since 1986, the IOC opened the Olympics up to "all the world's great male and female athletes," regardless of whether they received money for their sport. This change to the Olympic Charter effectively eliminated the 90-year-old ban on professional athletes, and the distinction between amateur and professional became much more blurred. In part, this change was precipitated by a growing consensus that sports was not only about personal honor and character, but also was a viable occupational option in which money, ambition, and personal marketing all played a necessary role. Under these modern circumstances, it is increasingly difficult to make a moral argument as it relates to sports.

THE INFLUENCE OF SPORTS AS AN ENTERTAINMENT INDUSTRY

As a matter of idealism, there is some measurable consensus on the value of genuinely enforcing anti-doping policies. As a practical matter, sports associations do not operate in a vacuum and idealism is often challenged by more pragmatic marketing interests. At the highest levels, professional and amateur sports make up a significant share of the entertainment industry, which requires sports associations to be responsive to public demand and other forces of market competition. Sports franchises must compete against each other and against other forms of entertainment for consumer dollars. The more action and drama associated with the sports, the more financial reward available to everyone associated with it. Typically, top tier athletes earn as much or more from endorsements than they do from their base salary, and the power of their endorsement is based almost exclusively on their ability to draw public attention and public support.

In recent years, athletes have been taking a larger share of the entertainment dollar than Hollywood film actors. In 2012, the top 10 highest paid athletes in the United States earned more at every rung than the top 10 actors. On average, the top 10 players earned $44 million a year from salary (or winnings) and endorsements, while the top 10 actors earned just over $36 million. Only musicians surpassed athletes in their portion of entertainment industry (with the top 10 musicians averaging $71 million). This was not the case a half century ago. In the 1950s, the average football player earned about $6,000 per season, which was a little more than twice the national average per household, but still much less than the $100,000–$300,000 paid out to actors per movie. The change in fortunes for sports players began in the 1970s as the players of major sports leagues began to form unions (also known as players' associations). By the 1980s, players associations in most sports earned the right to collective bargaining and, in several famous instances, they used strikes to compel franchise owners to guarantee minimum salaries and push for certain contract provisions. Baseball was the most active players association to exercise their collective bargaining options, resulting in eight strikes between 1972 and 1994. The last and most well-known strike of 1994–1995 resulted in a loss of the entire season.

By the late 1990s, the top athletes in the major sports (baseball, football, basketball) began to outearn their counterparts in Hollywood. The players associations gained leverage, in part, due to the rash of achievements and records broken during the 1990s. In baseball, the records for the most home runs earned in a single season set by Roger Maris in 1961 was broken six times by three different players between 1998 and 2001. Indeed, the pace of homeruns increased substantially. During the 70 years from 1920 to 1990, less than 10 people hit 50 homeruns or more in a single season, and during the nearly four decades that Maris's record held that milestone was reached by only three players. Yet, in the five years between 1996 and 2001, nine players managed to hit 50 homeruns or more on 15 separate occasions. The total number of homeruns hit per year by any player almost doubled throughout the 1990s, routinely reaching 5,500 or more. In Roger Maris's day, in 1961, the number of homeruns hit throughout the league had just surpassed 3,000 for the first time. Not surprisingly, the excitement generated by the rapid increase in hits led to significant increases in annual salaries and endorsement deals for baseball players. Also, not surprisingly, allegations of steroid use also increased.

The connection between steroid use and salary spikes is strongly correlated. Sports writers now call the late 1990s the steroid era because of the more than 120 baseball players who either admitted to using or were implicated by others as using hGH or other anabolic steroids. Six of the eight players who broke the 50 home run barrier, including the three players who broke Roger Maris's record (Barry Bonds, Sammy Sosa, and Mark McGuire) have all been implicated. Yet, despite the widespread public awareness of steroid use, the salaries and endorsement deals remain exceptionally high. In 2012, half of the top 50 highest paid athletes were baseball players. Moreover, almost all the athletes that have been implicated in doping scandals appear to be healthy—the only apparent penalties for their steroid use seem to be tarnished reputations.

For a young athlete making decisions based on the examples of their professional role models, the possible financial penalties (or risks) associated with getting caught taking ergogenic drugs does not appear to be as great as the prospective financial rewards (or benefits). Successful athletes achieve wealth, fame, and respectability far in excess of what might be expected by an ordinary occupation. If anabolic steroids seem to increase the likelihood of such success, then it is easy for a young person to overlook the accompanying risks to their physical and psychological health. The costs of doping are not easily demonstrated by their heroes who claim such a large percentage of media attention.

CHANCES OF TURNING PRO?

Unfortunately, the statistics taken from the successes (or scandals) of elite athletes do not tell the whole story. The National Collegiate Athletic Association reports that at any given time there are usually around 470,000 baseball players at the high school level, and of those only about 31,000 get to play at the college level. Yet, just a little more than 800 of these get recruited to play professional baseball each year—which adds up to a little more than half of 1 percent of all high school players. The numbers are even less hopeful in other sports. About 250 professional football players are drafted each year from a pool of about 67,000 college players, who in turn, come out of a group of 1.1 million high school athletes. Basketball has the lowest percentages, with more half a million high school players feeding just over 17,000 positions in college, out of which less than 50 professional positions are filled each year (adding up to 0.03% of all high school players). Despite these extremely small probabilities, the prospect of a professional career remains a popular dream for many young athletes.

Preprofessional Incentives—Economic and Cultural

The economic incentives for professional athletes may be the most obvious, but they are not unique in their efforts to combine competition with marketing needs. College athletes who demonstrate strong performance on winning teams are much more likely to be drafted to a professional team. Likewise, high school athletes who outshine their peers are much more likely to earn attractive college scholarships. At all levels, the pressure to succeed can reflect a mixture of old-fashioned competitiveness combined with an ambition for some degree of economic reward.

The dream of paying for college through sports is strong among both student athletes and their parents. In 2012, about $1 billion in athletic scholarships was awarded to graduating high school students. That number increases a little more than 4 percent each year. Unfortunately, the competition for that money remains tight. The percentage of students who receive athletic scholarships has been relatively constant since the 1980s, hovering somewhere between 1 and 2 percent. Also, according the National Collegiate Athletic Association (NCAA), the average athletic scholarship for sports such as swimming or track and field is about $2,000. For more revenue-generating sports like football and basketball, the average is a little more than $10,000. The average tuition, room, and board costs for a major university that is able to afford such scholarships ranges from $20,000 to $50,000 per year. A typical athletic scholarship will only cover about 15 percent of that total. Nevertheless, the prospects of potential benefits down the road often contribute to parent and student priorities from very early ages. A recent survey of coaches at NCAA Division I institutions indicates an increasing expectation among parents that athletic scholarships will cover all costs. The president of the NCAA, Myles Brand, confirmed the statistics, explaining, "The youth sports culture is overly aggressive, and while the opportunity for an athletic scholarship is not trivial, it's easy for the opportunity to be over exaggerated by parents and advisers."

Other cultural incentives contribute to the importance of participation in athletics at the high school level. Numerous studies published in the 1990s and 2000s show strong correlations that suggest students who participate in high school athletics are more likely to have fewer rates of discipline referrals, have higher grade point averages, and are more likely to move on to graduate from college than those who do not participate. Advisors often cite such studies to encourage students to pursue extracurricular sports-related activities.

Many of the studies that link student success with extracurricular involvement repeat the common conceptions held during the 1800s, which also linked amateur athletics to well-rounded character development.

There are other studies, however, from the 1990s and 2000s that distinguish between simple involvement and unique excellence. Research suggests that students that are most committed to athletics often have lower grade point averages and tend to value their athletic performance over their academic performance. The most competitive athletes often practice several hours a day, and there is little time for anything outside their sport. If students succeed in earning an athletic scholarship, the pressure only increases and the academic subjects tend to assume lesser concern. The eventual outcome of athletic excellence, then, seems to contradict the original more traditional appeal of extracurricular involvement. Critics, like Yesalis, argue that the original spirit of competition becomes corrupted by the external promises of future rewards, resulting in a single-minded focus on winning and achieving the next level of performance. Anabolic steroids and other ergogenic drugs magnify these cultural forces to create a self-reinforcing cycle leading to greater pressures for steroid use.

WADA AND USADA—THE SEARCH FOR INDEPENDENCE

Yesalis wrote *Anabolic Steroids in Sports and Exercise* in 1993, when the U.S. Congress had just recently reclassified anabolic steroids for nontherapeutic uses as a Schedule III controlled substance. At the time, both the National Football League (NFL) and the Major League Baseball (MLB) had anti-doping policies on paper, but there was reason to question whether professional sports associations were rigorously enforcing their own rules. Within a few years, the Tour de France was scandalized by the Festina incident on 1998, during which the coaches and trainers of numerous national teams were caught in possession of stockpiles of steroids and other ergogenic drugs. The following year, the IOC formed the World Anti-Doping Agency (WADA) in an attempt to create an association independent of the sports community, which would be charged with policing ergogenic drug use among athletes for all sports, free from economic, political, or cultural pressures. Though linked to the Olympic movement, one of the stated goals of WADA was to serve as the model for all sports federations and all national anti-doping programs, regardless of whether they are connected to the Olympics. In addition to the 168 sports associations reserved for athletes with disabilities (who play in the Paralympic Games), WADA also serves as the primary standard for 70 other international sports federations.

In 2000, the U.S. Olympic Committee organized its own independent association at the national level, called the U.S. Anti-Doping Agency (USADA). The obvious economic pressures faced by both the amateur and professional sports associations threatened the credibility of their internal anti-doping programs. The USADA is given sole responsibility for testing, adjudication, education, and research for the development of programs, policies, and procedures necessary to keep Olympic sports drug free. It adopts the WADA anti-doping code (called **the Code**) as its primary model. The USADA oversees most sports associated with the Olympic movement, but like WADA, the USADA hopes to set the standards for other national sports associations—including the professional leagues. Both WADA and USADA groups were formed out of recognition that the ideological incentives for drug-free sports are often overwhelmed by the pragmatic interests of modern sports culture.

USADA Guidelines

In 1967, when the IOC published its first list of banned substances, there were only five categories of substances and anabolic steroids were not included in the list. At the time, the list only banned substances that could be tested. Forty-five years later, in 2012, there were 13 categories of substances and medically enhanced training methods that are prohibited—some are prohibited at any time and others prohibited only during competition. WADA Code went into effect in 2004 and revised again in 2007 and 2013.

The list includes more than 200 specific chemical compounds, but it is not intended to be comprehensive. Within each subcategory, the list is preceded throughout with phrases that warn: the "list includes, but is not limited to" the following substances. These added qualifications are intended to cover future drugs that may not be included today, but which nevertheless violate the spirit of the prohibition. Almost since testing began, anti-doping officials recognized the race between scientists seeking new approaches to test for banned substances and those other scientists seeking new ergogenic drugs that are undetectable by the existing testing methods. To cover all contingencies, WADA and USADA list guidelines used in determining whether a substance should (or will) be included. Substances need only meet two of the three criteria to be included:

1. The drug or method has the potential to enhance sport performance.
2. It represents an actual or potential health risk to the athlete.
3. It violates the spirit of sport.

In addition, WADA and USADA also implemented certain procedures to ensure athletes were ergogenic drug free both in-season and off. During the 1970s and 1980s, athletes were often warned in advance when testing would occur, which meant that they could use ergogenic drugs out-of-competition, as long as there were no traces left before competition. That meant that athletes could train with steroids, and then end their use a certain number of weeks prior to the upcoming tests. To account for this possibility, Olympic athletes are currently subjected to random testing of both urine and blood samples at any day or time of the year and at any place. To accomplish this, WADA required all Olympic Athletes to submit the paperwork about their whereabouts that informed their regulating sports associations where they can be found at any time at three-month intervals.

In order to protect against designer steroids that might be difficult to detect, samples are stored for eight years. Athletes, who successfully evade detection through some advanced biochemical solution during one event, may face penalties five years later after the testing technology catches up with the evasion technology. One of the more famous examples of this was Lance Armstrong, who was caught blood doping years after his unprecedented string of seven consecutive Tour de France victories. At the time of his competition, blood doping was undetectable when players used their own stored blood because the chemical composition was exactly the same. In 2012, new technology was able to compare the RNA values within the blood sample to distinguish between fresh and stored blood.

The penalties for violating WADA and USADA anti-doping policies can be severe. Any athlete caught using ergogenic drugs will be stripped of any titles gained as a result of the doping, and barring some evidence to show that the drug use was accidental, the results of all other competitions during the event will also be disqualified. First violations result in a two-year suspension from competition and a second violation could result in a lifetime ban. Coaches, trainers, or others who supply drugs to players will also receive a ban of at least four years for a first offense and up to a lifetime ban depending on the severity. If drugs were supplied to a minor, the ban is for life. If an athlete fails to cooperate by missing a drug test or by failing to file paperwork indicating where they will be so that officials can find them to administer a random test, then the penalty could lead to one- or two-year bans. Failure to file appropriate **therapeutic use exemptions** prior to legitimate treatments may result in a failed test, and the athlete would be held responsible for the violation. Athletes are also responsible for any dietary and herbal supplements that may claim to be ergogenic free, yet still include banned substances. The WADA and USADA codes require athletes, their coaches, trainers, and other support staff to be informed, compliant, and prepared for testing at anytime and anyplace.

The WADA and USADA programs are intended to serve as institutional protections against the self-interest that is inherent in the sports industry.

Their jurisdiction, though, only applies to amateur and semiamateur sports associations. Professional sports associations, including the three majors NFL, MLB, and NBA, are not bound by WADA or USADA standards, except when individual athletes seek to compete in a WADA-sponsored event (like the Olympics). Since 1988, NBA players routinely compete in the Olympics and as such they are subject to the WADA Code. Outside of the Olympic competitions, the players return to the NBA anti-doping guidelines.

PROFESSIONAL SPORTS ASSOCIATIONS

At first glance, it would be easy to conclude that the major professional sports associations refuse to adhere to WADA and USADA anti-doping guidelines because they have a financial incentive for pursuing more lenient anti-doping procedures. There is little doubt that anabolic steroids improve player performance, and the higher the level of play the greater the public interest. Yet, the situation is complicated by the fact that most professional athletes belong to a players union, and as such the rules that regulate drug testing in the unionized workplace are subject to the National Labor Relations Act (NLRA). Athletes in the NFL, MLB, NBA, and NHL all rely on players unions to negotiate workplace conditions. Neither the employers nor the players unions may unilaterally make employment decisions, including choosing to adhere to WADA or USADA guidelines for anti-doping policies. Both sides must come to an agreement through collective bargaining. Since it is frequently not in the interest of either the owners or the players to rigorously enforce anti-doping rules, each side is free to blame the other for insincere implementation.

Among the three major professional sports associations, the NFL has been touted as the most comprehensive in its drug-testing policies. Like WADA and USADA codes, the NFL provides a list of banned substances, which players are potentially tested for year round. The program applies to players and other team personnel who work with players, including coaches and trainers. All players must be tested at least once per year, during the preseason, after which they are subject to random testing up to a maximum of 24 times per year (though, typically, individual players are tested with much less frequency). Tests are limited to urine samples, which can identify steroids levels but which cannot find hGH or other designer steroids. The NFL owners began discussing the possibility of blood tests in 2010, but no agreement was reached as of 2013. Penalties for drug violations range from a minimum four-game suspension for a first offence to an eight-game suspension for a second offence and a maximum one-year suspension for a third offence.

The NFL Standard

Compared to the MLB and the NBA, the NFL drug-testing program is more rigorous. The NBA only conducts drug tests during the training camp, and the MLB only tests during the season. Both the MLB and the NBA limit their testing to players, and do not include coaches, trainers, or other team personnel. Critics contend that the NBA policy allows players to use ergogenic drugs during the regular season with little risk of detection. The MLB tests all season, but there is room for players to use ergogenic drugs off season. Penalties for each are comparable, but none are as severe as those imposed by WADA or USADA. Also, for each professional sports association, the drug testing is conducted, and implemented in-house. There are no independent or outside associations like WADA or USADA monitoring the consistency of implementation.

In 2010, the *North Dakota Law Review* featured a Sports Law Symposium in which an article by Daniel Gandert and Fabian Ronisky argued that despite its rigorous reputation, the NFL anti-doping program was filled with loopholes that seriously undermined its credibility. First, the NFL system does not test players on the day of a game, which means that fast-acting steroids and other masking agents could potentially be used during competition and be flushed out of the system before the next random test. Second, although athletes are required to fill their urine specimen containers in the presence of a qualified official, there is also a provision that permits players to provide a makeup sample at a later time if they are unable to do so when requested. The makeup sample does not require a chaperone and may be submitted at a later time, which could allow unscrupulous players to substitute someone else's urine in place of their own with little risk of detection. Third, the NFL reserves the right to withhold positive test results from the public in order to protect the player privacy. In practice, such scandal protection could permit the industry to escape popular pressures for clean games. These examples suggest that the strength of an anti-doping policy cannot be judged by the codified guidelines alone. The practical implementation of the testing procedures may reveal loopholes that undermine the policy intent.

Gandert and Ronisky argued that the drug policies of American professional sports associations were fundamentally flawed because they relied on labor standards and not the standards established by the global anti-doping movement. This criticism could be applied to any sports association that involves players unions. There is potential for legal loopholes unforeseen by either the owners or the players. For example, in 2008, two players from the Minnesota Vikings used the peculiar laws of their state to challenge decisions made by an NFL policy administered out of state.

After failing a drug test, Pat Williams and Kevin Williams claimed they unknowingly ingested the steroid-masking agents at their homes and were thus protected by the laws of their home state, which prevents employment penalties for drugs taken outside the workplace. After two and a half years, the courts eventually decided in favor of the NFL, but the precedent of similar future challenges remain when the basis for the policies are based on laws that were not intended to serve athletic associations.

Since the creation of the USADA in 2000, lawmakers have routinely submitted bills that would force all professional sports associations to adopt the same anti-doping policies as WADA and USADA. At every congressional session, the bills are referred to a committee but fail to garner much support. In theory, the federal government has the authority to regulate national sports teams under the Commerce Clause. In 1957, the Supreme Court ruled in *Radovich v. National Football League* that professional leagues operate in interstate commerce, and a later ruling of *Flood v. Kuhn* (1972) held that drug testing of interstate businesses could be regulated by the Congress. In practice, however, there is serious question as to whether the Congressional right to regulate interstate businesses supersedes union protections guaranteed under the NLRA. Gandert and Ronisky argue they do. Other attorneys for the players associations would argue to the contrary.

COLLEGIATE AND HIGH SCHOOL ASSOCIATIONS

Perhaps, the group that continues to represent Pierre de Coubertin vision of amateur athletes is the student players in both the high school and collegiate levels. In order to participate in the NCAA Division I and II competitions, students must complete a certificate of amateurism that verifies they have not received compensation directly or indirectly for their sport. Amateur athletes may not enter into an agreement to be represented by an agent, they may not tryout, practice, or compete with a professional team, and they may not delay their college enrollment in order to participate in organized sports. This not only includes limitations on the kinds of events that students may participate in, but it also limited the amount of financial aid and other forms of support that the universities may offer as recruitment incentives. In addition to amateur status, students must also graduate from high school and earn and maintain minimum grade point averages. In part, the purpose for the NCAA eligibility restrictions is to ensure that students devote at least some part of their attention to academics while they attend school. In part, also, the purpose of amateur status is to protect the integrity of the playing field by ensuring that each student athlete is protected from an overly market-oriented sports environment.

The NCAA drug-testing program began in 1986, with testing at championship events. By 1990, the program expanded to include year-round testing of athletes competing in Division I and II schools. In addition, most participating universities include their own drug-testing programs that generally adhere to NCAA standards. Universities do not have to report their findings to NCAA, but they must be consistent in their policies or risk sanctions, including suspensions from NCAA events. Unlike the standards set by either WADA or the professional sports associations, the likelihood of multiple drug tests for student athletes is relatively low. More than 430,000 student athletes participate in NCAA sports programs, and of those approximately 11,000 will be randomly tested in all sports. Players who make it to the championship levels will be tested more frequently than those who do not.

Since the student athletes must also abide by the standards of conduct set by the university, NCAA drug tests include ergogenic drugs as well as common street drugs that may have no performance-enhancing effects. The categories of banned substances include stimulants, alcohol and beta blockers, masking agents (such as diuretics), peptide hormones, antiestrogens and Beta-2 Agonists, and street drugs (such as marijuana, cocaine, or heroin). Tests are administered by officials from both NCAA and member schools. The penalties for failed drug tests are similar to those set by WADA and USADA programs. First violations for either ergogenic or street drugs result in a one-year ineligibility. Students who fail a second test for street drugs lose a second year of eligibility. Those who fail a second test for ergogenic drugs will be permanently ineligible.

The amateur status of student athletes means there is no overlapping jurisdiction between NCAA rules and the anti-doping policies of professional sports associations. There is, however, some overlap with WADA and USADA for student athletes who compete in Olympic events.

Legality of High School Drug Testing

As the age of the student athlete lowers, the expectations and responsibilities of the sports associations become more complicated. Prior to the 1980s, random drug testing among middle and high school students was unheard of. Recreational drug use among teens was most problematic during the 1970s, when reports of illicit drug use among high school seniors averaged around 50 percent (including anything from marijuana, to cocaine, to heroine, and amphetamines). At the time, most parents and school officials presumed that random drug tests violated student's guaranteed constitutional rights of unwarranted search and seizure. By the end of the decade, however, drug-control advocates argued that students in a school setting fell under an exception to the Fourth Amendment protections reserved for administrative searches.

During the 1980s, the elder President George Bush launched a war on drugs that targeted youth education and intervention. Most schools adopted a zero-tolerance policy, which included automatic expulsion for possession of drugs on campus, and most states increased mandatory minimum sentencing requirements for dealers who sold drugs within a certain distance of a schoolyard. Many schools installed metal detectors to screen for guns, and drug-sniffing dogs were allowed to pass by the lockers to check for drugs (reactions from the dogs outside the locker constituted probable cause to search inside the locker).

The rates of illicit drug use among high school students decreased, with averages of 40 percent among high school seniors in the early 1980s, decreasing to a low of just under 30 percent in 1992. The increased sensitivity to drug abuse among youth, combined with the increasing levels of intervention routinely employed by schools with histories of drug abuse, opened the way for more expanded drug-testing policies for student athletes. In 1988, a school district in Indiana launched a program that randomly tested student athletes for drugs—focusing mostly on common street drugs. The parents of two students sued claiming their children's rights were violated by unwarranted searches. The school district argued that they had an obligation to ensure a safe environment and that they had a history of drug problems. Moreover, they explained that all students signed waivers agreeing to the conditions prior to participating and the penalties of a failed drug test resulted in referrals to counseling and not expulsion from school.

The case reached the U.S. Supreme Court *Schaill v. Tippecanoe* (1988), which held that participation in high school athletics was a privilege and not a right. Therefore, students who voluntarily participate are subject to reduced expectations of privacy. Later, the Court affirmed the right of schools districts to require suspicionless drug tests of all student athletes in *Vernonia School District v. Acton* (1995), because students had a lower expectation of privacy at school, and because drugs threatened the safety of student athletes. Last, in 2002, the Supreme Court ruled in *Earls v. Tecumseh Public School District* that schools could require drug testing of any student involved in any extracurricular activity, whether the activity was sports related or not. The decreased expectation of privacy for students, combined with the relatively noninvasive urinalysis testing procedures, meant that the school "was entirely reasonable" in enacting a drug-testing policy as a means of protecting student safety and health.

State High School Sports Associations

During the 1990s and 2000s, the decision to implement drug-testing policies for middle and high school students was left to each individual school district. Usually, the costs of implementing the program were weighed against the perceived magnitude of the illicit drug problem in the local area. Standard tests for common street drugs (marijuana, cocaine, amphetamines, etc.) could range from $15 to $30 per student, while more intensive tests for anabolic steroids could be as expensive as $200 for each player.

The public pressure to protect students from the increasingly poor examples demonstrated by professional athletes intensified after Drug Enforcement Agency (DEA) agents raided the Bay Area Laboratory Co-Operative headquarters in 2003 and discovered a network of scientists and doctors who provided designer steroids for elite athletes. The scandal implicated dozens of professional athletes, including the baseball player, Barry Bonds, who had earlier broken records for most home runs hit in a single season. Concerned parents across the country began calling for more systematic and uniform drug-testing policies for all student athletes. In 2004, the younger President George W. Bush included a statement in his State of the Union Address that called on "team owners, union representatives, coaches and players to take the lead, to send the right signal, to get tough and to get rid of steroids now." Senate hearings were held for the next four years, which included testimonies for dozens of current and former professional players who admitted or denied steroid use.

The effort captured national attention, leading to a broad pressure for professional sports to enact more meaningful anti-doping programs that were similar to the standard established by WADA and the USADA. Though the response was unevenly applied, the NFL, MLB, and the NHL publicly supported the effort to protect youth against the dangers of anabolic steroid abuse. Together, the associations contributed money to numerous advocacy groups, including the Taylor Hooten Foundation, which was established in 2004 by Don Hooten and his wife after the suicide of their 17-year-old son, which they attribute to his use of anabolic steroids. The Hooten Foundation began lobbying state lawmakers to be more assertive in their oversight of high school athletic programs. The *Earls* decision affirmed the legality of random drug tests among middle and high school students, so the only major drawback to broad implementation was funding.

In 2006, New Jersey became the first state to implement statewide anti-doping policies that included random drug tests for high school students.

The New Jersey State Interscholastic Athletic Association spent $400,000 to test 2,000 students. Two years later, in 2008, Florida launched a similar program, with a $100,000 budget that tested 600 students. Texas, the home of the Taylor Hooten Foundation, followed suit the same year with the nation's largest steroid-testing program, with a budget of $3 million to test 19,000 students. By contrast, the NCAA administers less than 16,000 tests a year. Illinois passed a similar program the following year on a smaller scale and funded directly by the athletes, without requiring taxpayers support. Meanwhile, debates among lawmakers waged in West Virginia, New Mexico, Connecticut, Delaware, Louisiana, and California.

After a few years, all but two of the programs were terminated. In part, the success of the drug-testing programs was difficult to measure, and therefore the continued funding was difficult to sustain. In Florida, there was only one failed test among the 600 administered. New Jersey also resulted in one failed test out of 500. In Texas, there were seven failed tests out of 19,000. The 12 athletes (out of a pool of 1,000) which failed tests

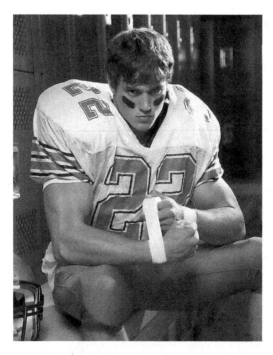

Without clear data on the levels of steroid abuse in youth sports, some activists think more states should follow the lead of New Jersey, which in 2007 became the first state to adopt a program of mandatory testing for high school athletes. (Dreamstime.com)

in Illinois were all later cleared by the state medical review officers. As a result, lawmakers in Florida ended the program and the state legislature eventually reduced the Texas program down to $750,000 in 2010. Opponents of the program argued that the drug tests were ineffective because they did not include most modern steroids and that they were limited to easily defining time periods during the sports seasons, which made them easy to evade. Advocates for the program contended that the purpose of drug testing was not to catch users, but to deter students from using it in the first place. The required paperwork and drug-testing procedures provided a vehicle for parents, coaches, and other influences to explain the physical, psychological, and ethical dangers associated with anabolic steroids. Ultimately, the debate focused around priorities. As Don Hooten explained, "They can talk about the costs of the tests all they want [but] Plano [Texas] just built a $20 million football facility. . . . They have the money; it's just an unwillingness to spend it elsewhere."

Students with No Association Affiliation

For a time after 2011, the trend of state-mandated drug testing for high school athletes began to wane. The economic downturn combined with the mixed perceptions of efficacy prompted many states to reduce or cancel funding. The momentum shifted, though, in 2013 after another laboratory in Florida was revealed to have supplied designer steroids to elite and amateur athletes alike. The Biogenesis Medical and Wellness Center described itself as an antiaging clinic, but its client lists included more than a dozen professional baseball players (including Alex Rodriguez), and nearly as many high school and college student athletes. Immediately following the disclosure, the Florida High School Athletic Association formed a panel to look into new approaches to drug testing, which might include greater emphasis on coaches and adult employees who may contribute to the distribution of ergogenic drugs and the evasion of drug tests. The Hooten Foundation added that their new approach would combine education with interdiction. As Don Hooten explained, "Unless you're doing Olympic-quality testing, you'll never catch all the cheaters—and we know that's just not economically feasible for most of the school districts out there." He added, "The threat of testing combined with an effective education effort has the best chance of preventing this from spreading."

Despite the low numbers of failed drug tests, the evidence suggests the number of middle and high school students taking anabolic steroids is relatively high. According to a survey conducted by the University of Minnesota, over 1.5 million teens admit to using steroids, and the medium age for first time steroid use was 15. The rate of abuse seems to be increasing. The Center for Disease Control and Prevention (CDC) estimated the rate of users in 1993 was 1 out of 45 high school students. Five years later, the rate increased almost twice to 1 out of 27 students. In 2013, the rate was estimated to be 1 out of 16. Anabolic steroid use is twice as common as illicit use of hard drugs such as methamphetamines, inhalants, heroin, or cocaine, but only slightly less commonly used than marijuana.

CRACK DEALERS VERSUS STEROIDS DEALERS?

Drug dealers target youthful steroid users in much the same way as they would other drugs. In 2011, drug enforcement agents uncovered a 32-member drug ring that sold to youths near a local YMCA in Ohio. Officials found more than $600,000 in steroids imported from China and confiscated $300,000 in cash and a wide assortment of assault rifles, semiautomatic pistols, shotguns, and ammunition. The network spanned several counties and two states, but seemed to be targeting mostly high school-aged teens.

Reports from the CDC also indicate that boys are more likely than girls to use steroids (5.9% of boys compared to 4.6% of girls). The disparity may be due to the fact that most students do not use ergogenic drugs for sports-related competition. Almost two-thirds of teens say they take anabolic steroids to improve their looks—girls want to lose weight and boys want to gain muscle. This also accounts for the high percentage (35%) of students who take protein powders and other muscle-enhancing supplements that are legally sold over the counter (often including images of muscular men and perfectly toned women on the labels).

Most dietary supplements are not regulated by the FDA, and could potentially trigger a failed drug test for WADA, USADA, and NCAA levels of analysis. The most common supplements are whey protein, creatine, and **dehydroepiandrosterone** (DHEA). DHEA is naturally produced in the body, though levels gradually decrease with age. It is used as an antiaging supplement intended to restore energy and maintain bone mass. It is legally sold over the counter, but as a precursor to anabolic steroids, it is banned by WADA, USADA, and NCAA. **Creatine** is also naturally produced in the body and is used as a supplement to increase **adenosine triphosphate** levels, providing muscles with more energy to build and repair themselves. It can lead to fluid retention and may interfere with the kidney function but is otherwise legal for over-the-counter drug sales.

Neither creatine nor **whey proteins** are included on the list of prohibited substances, but they may potentially contain other additives that may trigger a failed drug test. The Taylor Hooten Foundation contends that such supplements contribute to a chemical culture that promotes artificial expectations of body image and encourages physical beauty over internal character development as a primary measure of self-worth.

Education efforts that target teen anabolic steroid abuse are complicated by the diverse motivation behind the use. Studies used by the Taylor Hooten Foundation indicate that the top three reasons for steroid use among teens are: (1) to improve their physical appearance; (2) to feel better about themselves; and (3) to improve athletic performance. Athletes who turn to steroids in their high school years stand a fair chance of facing some level of intervention from a related sports association, including the local high school district, their future NCAA University, and potentially WADA or USADA if they seek Olympic levels of competition. For those other students who take steroids for cosmetic reasons and who are not subject to any local, state, or national association oversight, the chances for interdiction are much lower.

Moral Corruption of the Youth

Historically, public pressure to regulate and police ergogenic drug use is strongly tied to fears of the cultural impact on the physical, psychological, and moral development of youth. National scandals that tie certain professional and elite amateur athletes with anabolic steroids may not directly involve teens, but critics fear that as role models these athletes potentially send the message that anabolic steroids are unavoidable—perhaps, even necessary—elements for competitive success. The Taylor Hooten Foundation would argue that these messages undermine the moral health of the culture by emphasizing external standards of self-fulfillment (physical beauty, fame, material wealth) rather than those intrinsic values that are more enduring and are less likely to fade over time. In their public statements, these sentiments are repeated by representatives of the players associations of the NFL, MLB, NBA, and NHL, as well as the representatives of team and franchise owners. Public discussion may question the utility of drug testing or the relative threshold of personally acceptable risk for professional and elite-level athletes, but there is very little debate over whether teenage youth should be using anabolic steroids for anything other than therapeutic purposes. The vast majority of discussions related to teen drug use involve questions about how best to end the problem.

OTHER NON-SPORTS-RELATED ASSOCIATIONS

Nontherapeutic uses of anabolic steroids are most often associated with performance enhancement for competition, though teens and celebrities are most often motivated by cosmetic reasons. There are a few kinds of associations outside the realm of competitive sports that also try to regulate the use of ergogenic drugs. Their influence is perhaps less noticeable, but they still play a role in influencing the trends and priorities of popular culture.

Professional Wrestling

Professional wrestlers fit into a category that combines sports and entertainment. The participants compete for public appeal, but the outcomes of the events are more often scripted or predetermined than a reflection of a balanced contest. Professional wrestlers are typically hired under contract by a national or regional franchise who organizes competitions for live, televised, or recorded events. Two of the largest professional wrestling associations are World Wrestling Entertainment (WWE) and Total Non-Stop Action Wresting (TNA), and though they each have drug-testing policies in place, there is little enforcement.

Public attention generally recognizes professional wrestling as belonging to a different category of athletes as football, baseball, or basketball players, and there are few calls for WADA or USADA type standards for participation. Instead, the professional wrestlers are usually equated with performers and actors, and the steroid use is more for cosmetic purposes than performance enhancement. Since the outcomes are largely predetermined, the primary purpose behind the massive muscle bulk is to create an impressive image for the attending audience. The Screen Actors Guild does not have a steroid policy and there is no public demand to establish one.

Nevertheless, anabolic steroids for nontherapeutic purposes are illegal, and an organization that knowingly and repeatedly conspires to break federal law is liable to charges under the Racketeer Influenced Corrupt Organizations Act of 1970. No cases have been filed under the statute except in situations related to steroids trafficking and distribution. Nevertheless, the WWE association established a steroids-testing program in the early 1990s shortly after they were reclassified as a Schedule III controlled substance. There was no evidence that the program was actually implemented, and the CEO Vince McMahon eliminated the program in 1996 with an explanation that the "incidence of illegal and performance enhancing drugs is so slight that group testing is no longer cost effective or necessary."

Public opinion began to change in 2005 after WWE wrestler Eddie Guerrero died in his hotel room at the age of 38. He had a history of drug abuse, which included cocaine. Autopsy results indicated Guerrero suffered from arteriosclerotic heart disease, which means his blood vessels were not supplying enough oxygen to his heart, which had enlarged after years of steroid abuse. Two weeks before his death, Guerrero had been given prescriptions for nandrolone, testosterone, and anastrozole (which is used to counter water retention and breast enlargement that usually accompanies steroid use). The media attention forced McMahon to institute a new drug-testing program for WWE wrestlers in 2006. After the first year, 40 percent of the wrestlers tested positive despite preannounced warnings.

The following year, another WWE wrestler Chris Benoit murdered his wife and son before committing suicide. His testosterone levels were 10 times the normal level, which prompted a Senate investigation into steroid use in professional wrestling. Around the same time, DEA agents raided Florida pharmacy, Signature Pharmacy, for selling anabolic steroids over the internet to consumers without a prescription. During the raid, the names of more than a dozen WWE wrestlers were included in the prescription list. WWE suspended dozens of wrestlers, but it did not prevent them from competing in televised events or in live performances. Benoit had been tested four times for anabolic steroids and failed three of them, yet he received no suspensions or other penalties.

The public showed no signs of surprise following these revelations, because the expectations of performers are not the same as the standards held for elite athletes in genuinely competitive sports. Nevertheless, the Senate Oversight Committee responsible for the hearings recommended some regulatory action to deal with the widespread steroid use by professional wrestlers. The reason, as committee Chair Henry Waxman explained, was because "over 3 million children and teenagers watch professional wrestling each year. The apparently widespread use of steroids in professional wrestling sends the wrong message to youth." No legislation followed Waxman's recommendation, mostly because the public did not express strong support for the action.

Police Officers

Unlike the WWE or TNA entertainment associations, both the labor unions and administrative hierarchies associated with law enforcement and other first responders take the issue of anabolic steroids abuse very seriously. Public concern over steroid abuse within ranks is more difficult to measure. Law enforcement officers and firefighters place their lives at risk on a daily basis, and public support for that commitment is very high. When evidence surfaces of ergogenic drug use within these groups, public reaction is usually mixed.

In 2008, the lead article in the International Association of Police Chiefs monthly magazine, *The Police Chief*, highlighted the potential problem of anabolic steroid use and abuse among police officers. In addition to news stories of baseball stars, Olympic athletes, and elite athletes who were embarrassed or stripped of their titles as a result of their ergogenic drug use, headlines also reported raids of internet pharmacies and antiaging clinics that included names of police officers and firefighters among their client lists. A few years earlier, a single raid on the Florida-based PowerMedica implicated 14 officers who had recently purchased hGH and other anabolic steroids. The authors of the article warned that unless the issue was confronted directly, the future may be one where they "look back on what could be an embarrassing 'steroid era' of law enforcement—one in which the profession might be riddled with lawsuits, corruption, and claims of heavy-handedness." To avoid this situation, the article recommended increased education efforts for both officers and administrators, drug-testing programs based on reasonable cause, and a penalty of automatic administrative leave pending further investigation for any failed tests.

One difficulty facing administrative officials is that most safety enforcement personnel are unionized. As such, they fall under many of the same complexities that impact the professional sports players associations, since drug testing in the workplace usually falls under the NLRB Act. The Supreme Court ruled in the *National Treasury Employees Union v. Von Raab* (1989) that employees carrying firearms could be required to submit to drug testing. Yet, two years later, the Massachusetts State Supreme Court struck down random drug policy set in place by the Boston Police Department as a violation of collective bargaining rules. Actual application of internal drug-testing programs varies greatly from state to state and from department to department. In many cases, testing is limited by budgetary concerns since steroid tests are up to 10 times more expensive than tests for standard street drugs.

By 2012, investigations in Oregon, Ohio, Michigan, Indiana, New York, and New Jersey implicated hundreds of police officers. In New Jersey, one drug bust implicated 248 public safety officials after a local newspaper *Ledger-Star* ran a three-part series on the "secret world of steroid use by law enforcement." New Jersey's attorney general followed the recommendation presented earlier by the International Association of Police Chiefs, and the largest New Jersey police union supported random drug testing, as long as local departments maintained discretion over how or when to implement it since some local budgets might not be able to afford the costs. The greatest fear among both the administrators and the officers was that rumors of widespread steroid abuse might lead to unsubstantiated charges of brutality anytime an officer used force in apprehending a suspect.

Firefighters and Soldiers

Public expectations of steroid-free police officers are somewhat different from their expectations for firefighters. Both branches involve public service, and both require physical fitness, which may pressure members to seek ergogenic drugs to help facilitate. Nevertheless, the public reaction to news stories of firefighters involved in steroid drug busts was more tempered. A 2013 story covering a scandal implicating six firefighters in Marietta, Georgia, drew some mixed reactions. Some argued that firefighters should be held to the same standard as any common citizen. Others argued that the need for enhanced performance may be the critical difference in saving someone's life. Unlike police officers, there is generally little fear of firefighters abusing their positions of authority. As one resident wrote, "If I was in a fire, I'd want the biggest strongest fireman available to pull me and my family out."

Public expectations for soldiers are similarly mixed. There is a great deal of support for soldiers and their willingness to place themselves in harm's way for the sake of protecting their country. At the same time, because they carry guns there is also some public concern that the risks of overly aggressive behavior could lead to unnecessary dangers both for soldiers and civilians. The official statistics of anabolic steroid abuse released by the Department of Defense are likely a little low since admission of use under the Uniform Code of Military Justice could result in a reduction of rank or expulsion from the military. A 2005 survey indicated 1.5 percent of soldiers illegally used anabolic steroids and a 2008 survey indicated a 2.5 percent usage rate. Yet, in 2009, an investigation of infantry units at an Army base near Seattle led to reports of 50 percent of more soldiers preparing to depart for field assignments in the Middle East use ergogenic drugs as part of the training regimen.

The official position of the Army is strict prohibition of anabolic steroids for ergogenic purposes. General Peter Chiarelli, the Army's vice chief of staff, explained, "The use of steroids is a short-term gain for long-term problems that individuals are going to have, and we cannot tolerate them in any way, shape, or form." Yet, the Army's broadly applied random drug-testing program does not include testing for steroids. Only a few hundred soldiers are tested for steroids as compared to the 450,000 tests for street drugs (marijuana, cocaine, and narcotics). From the perspective of infantry troops, the expectation of steroid use is much different. One report quoted an Army Ranger who admitted using steroids while in Iraq. He recognized the side effects of increased aggressiveness and emotional highs and lows, but he explained, "There is a broad spectrum of things that could kill you in a war zone. You need to be aggressive and quick. I would do them again in a heartbeat."

The dangers of overaggressiveness in the field could be counterproductive to war aims and can trigger strong public reactions. In 2012, Staff Sergeant Robert Bales was stationed in Afghanistan when he got drunk and broke away from the camp in the middle of the night and went from house to house eventually killing 16 civilians and wounding 6 others. During his court martial the following year, he claimed that the combination of alcohol and steroid abuse led to the outburst. He pled guilty to the murders in exchange for avoiding the death penalty. Though many critics used the incident to call for withdrawal of troops overseas, there were few calls for more rigorous anti-doping policies. Both supporters and opponents of the war effort recognized the violent nature of the military environment, though they differ on the best solution for limiting unintended civilian casualties. For both sides of the argument, the role of anabolic steroids was not considered as significant a factor to Bales's crime as were the pressures of his immediate environment.

Animals for Racing and Related Competitions

There is a long historical precedent for drug-testing policies for animals used in racing and other performance-related competitions. In fact, prohibitions against doping horses predated rules against doping humans by 25 years, and effective drug-testing policies for animals emerged more than 50 years before those developed for humans. For the most part, these precautions grew out of the gambling culture associated with animal racing, and the testing protocols were motivated by a desire to ensure even playing fields. Yet, even in the 19th century, the gambling interests were accompanied by some concerns for the humane treatment of animals—particularly for horses. In the contemporary era, associations governing animal sports rely on the same two justifications for anti-doping policies as those associations governing humans: (1) protect the safety of the player (animal welfare concerns) and (2) protect the integrity of the sport (even playing field).

Horse sports, including various racing events, are included among the summer Olympic Games. As such, WADA sets the standards for drug-testing protocols for both human and animal competitors. Just as with traditional human sports, animals are randomly tested for a variety of prohibited substances, with automatic tests for winners of each event. Unlike their human companions, the animals are not tested off-season, so there is no need for quarterly notifications of animal whereabouts. Also, the list of prohibited substances is slightly different, with different standards of measurement. Since 1988, a research group from the University of Kentucky introduced a highly sensitive testing method called the **enzyme-linked immunosorbent assay** (ELISA), which requires only a drop of the animal's urine to determine quickly the presence of a prohibited substance. A positive indication then triggers a second more precise test using gas or liquid chromatography with mass spectrometry, which is the standard procedure used for human athletes.

The categories of prohibited ergogenic drugs include stimulants, tranquilizers, bronchodilators, and behavioral modifiers. Anabolic steroids are prohibited, but they are not commonly associated with improved race performance. Most European racing associations ban anabolic steroids for horses, but other regions only ban the drugs on game day. The trainer of the 2008 Kentucky Derby winner, Rick Dutrow, admitted he injected his horse Big Brown with anabolic steroids, which at the time was not prohibited. Steroids were treated as therapeutic drugs in the United States, but the perception of foul play was so great that many local race clubs prohibited its use for game day competitions. In 2013, a trainer from the United Arab Emirates was banned from British racing for eight years after his horse tested positive, which prompted the International Federation of Horse Racing Authorities to consider a global ban.

In most cases, catabolic steroids are seen to be more effective in performance enhancing because they help to decrease inflammations and in some cases open up airways (bronchodilators), which can have a significant impact on an animal's endurance. Since animals are not tested outside of competition, trainers often use a variety of antibiotics, anti-inflammatories, and anesthetic painkillers to enable more frequent training regimens with quicker healing times. If administered by a certified veterinarian for therapeutic purposes, these methods are legal and permissible under WADA guidelines, as long as all traces of the drug are metabolized back to normally expected levels prior to the competition (called **thresholds**). These therapeutic use exceptions are measured in much the same way that testosterone is measured in humans—the naturally occurring chemicals must be limited to the levels expected in nontreated animals. For all other nontherapeutic drugs, WADA maintains a **zero-tolerance** policy, which means even trace amounts will result in a failed test.

As with the human sports, WADA standards are used as the model guidelines for international associations (such as the International Federation for Equestrian Sports) and national and local associations (such as U.S. Equestrian Federation or the New York Jockey Club). In addition, because gambling is involved, each state establishes their own anti-doping policies through state gaming commissions, which regulate horse and dog racing. These almost always adhere to WADA standards. Unlike the human sports, there is no professional analogue to horse racing associations that operate independently from these traditional associations.

Drug-testing guidelines for dog racing associations are slightly different. Since greyhound dog racing is also tied directly to gambling, they are regulated by state-based gaming commissions in much the same way as horse racing. The categories of prohibited drugs and therapeutic thresholds are also mostly similar, with the notable exception that anabolic steroids are routinely used on female dogs as an estrus inhibitor, which works as a form of birth control. Female dogs usually receive monthly injections throughout the duration of their racing career (usually three or four years) to prevent them from going into heat. This practice is not unique to race dogs, and is commonly used for household pets and show animals for the same purpose. There is no evidence that these treatments enhance performance. Some animal rights activists contend that the anabolic steroid injections can result in liver damage, genital infections, and increased aggressiveness. Despite a few local prohibitions, the practice remains common nationally and WADA standards view the anabolic injections as a therapeutic use exception. There are no dog-related sports in the Olympics yet, but the International Federation of Sleddog Sports (IFSS) has been working with WADA since 2007 in an attempt to introduce sled dog events to the winter Olympic games. The IFSS drug-testing program follows the basic template used by the horse racing associations.

Steroid Hormones for Animal Growth (and Human Consumption)

The Food and Drug Administration (FDA) works in tandem with the U.S. Department of Agriculture and other state and federal regulatory bodies to ensure the safety of agricultural products before they reach the consumer. The FDA was the first federal agency developed to ensure consumer protection, and remains the cornerstone of other related agencies. In addition, industrial associations, such as the American Dairymen Association or the U.S. Farmers & Ranchers Alliance (USFRA), also establish guidelines for their members that ensure adherence to state and federal standards.

Anabolic steroids occur naturally in both animals and humans in the form of estradiol, progesterone, and testosterone. Beef producers use endogenous (naturally occurring forms) of anabolic steroids at low doses to promote tissue growth in animals. These steroids are usually marketed as pellets, which are injected into the cow's ear just below the skin to deliver low doses throughout the life of the animal. The FDA determined that the doses are so low that they only impact the growth of muscle tissue and do not result in elevated levels of anabolic hormones beyond what would ordinarily be expected in animal tissues. As such, the FDA approves the use of endogenous anabolic steroids for food-producing animals. Synthetic forms of anabolic steroids, such as trenbolone acetate, zeranol, and melengestrol acetate, exhibit slower metabolic rates and are only approved for defined doses to ensure that traces of the hormones remain the same as that which would be expected from untreated animals of the same age and sex.

In addition to anabolic steroids, farmers and ranchers also rely on a wide variety of antibiotics and protein hormones to ensure more consistent animal health, growth, and resource production in the shortest amount of time. Some of these include Bovine Growth Hormone (BGH), which is the cattle equivalent of hGH and is used to increase milk production. Each chemical supplement must be approved by the FDA before use and evidence of deliberate regulatory violations could result in significant civil repercussions. The FDA does not, however, closely monitor marketing terms and the phrase organic as it relates to meats, only refers to the fact that the animals did not receive added antibiotics or growth hormones. It does not mean that the products are free of endogenous hormone levels.

Some critics contend that the use of antibiotics and hormones (both steroid and protein based) undermine the general health of the consumers. In the 1950s, farmers used to add antibiotics in animals to promote tissue growth, but by the 1960s the FDA restricted the use of antibiotics for therapeutic purposes (to treat specific disease threats) or subtherapeutic levels (as inoculants for nonspecific disease threats.) The primary threat of overusing antibiotics is that it might lead to more drug resistant bacterial populations. The FDA has not been able to establish a pathway between bacterial resistance in livestock and those found in humans, though critics argue the pathway is undiscovered and not nonexistent. The fear of BGH and other anabolic steroids is that they may lead to the same kinds of ailments that are linked to human use of such drugs, including premature sexual development, enhanced sensitivity to allergens, and increased cancer risks. Though no clinical studies had uncovered a causal or correlational connection between the hormone-treated foods and these health risks, critics would argue that the discoveries are still to be made.

For its part, the FDA stands by its scientific research, which indicates that steroid-enhanced and BGH-treated food is chemically no different than the untreated foods. The USFRA association also argues that the use of hormones (steroid and protein based) helps produce healthier, leaner, and more abundant meat resulting in reduced environmental impact. Each pound of meat produced since 2007 uses 19 percent less feed, 33 percent less land, 12 percent less water, and 9 percent less fuel than what was required in 1977. In addition, the dairy farmers require almost 80 percent fewer animals to produce the same amount of milk than was required in 1944. The USFRA also notes that most animals do not use anabolic steroids. Although 95 percent of cattle use supplemental hormones for beef production, only 15 percent of cows in the United States use hormones to increase milk production. No hormones are used to increase growth for pork or poultry.

In many cases, the public debate over the use of anabolic steroids and growth hormones in animals for food production is influenced by the concurrent education efforts to warn students and athletes about the dangers of ergogenic drugs for sport. From a clinical perspective, the two uses are not related. From the perspective of cultural priorities, the connection is small. Those who fear about the dangers of a dominant chemical culture are also most likely to be concerned about the use of hormones in agricultural products.

Steroids for Show Animals

The drug policies of most associations that oversee sport and food-bearing animals focus on concerns related to an equal playing field and the health and safety of the animals. Their attention is concentrated on the conditions of the animal and not on the cultural risks that the animal's ergogenic drug use might pose for their handler. This is not true for animal-related associations that work most closely with youth. The exhibition of animals for county and state fairs are usually regulated by a combination of policies devised by the local venue and a related state or national association, such as the 4-H or Future Farmers of America youth organizations. Though the safety of animals and handlers remain of primary importance followed by assurance of fair competition, the other objective is to provide an educational and meaningful experience for the youth. In some ways, this last objective is the most compelling motivation for drug-testing policies in youth livestock shows.

Unlike the racing and sport animals, the drug testing of show stock is much more comprehensive. The top animals in each category are later auctioned off for sale as a carcass. Since the buyers are often strong sup-porters of youth competitions, the prices may be substantially higher than market value. In 2005, a 13-year-old girl sold her champion steer at a Texas Stock Show for $151,000. In 2002, another Texan steer was sold for $135,000. Average prices in local county fairs can often bring in thou-sands of dollars. After the auction, the animal is butchered and the carcass is tested for illegal drugs, chemicals, or feed additives before the meat is released to the buyer (and the money and awards released to the competi-tor). Therapeutic use exceptions exist for show animals as they do for the racing associations, but the list of prohibited substances is less defined. There is little concern for ergogenic drugs that impact speed or endurance, but competitors may be tempted to use chemicals, drugs, or other artificial means to change the appearance of the animals or make them behave more appropriately during exhibition. The general rule is that no animals should be given supplements that would not otherwise be approved by the FDA for animals destined for human consumption. Similar to WADA standards, the exhibitor is held responsible for any chemicals that might be found in the animal carcass.

The high prices that emerge during livestock shows may motivate some parents to pursue unethical means of securing victory for their son or daughter. Variants of anabolic steroids may be used to increase muscle mass in select locations, while variants of catabolic steroids may be applied elsewhere to reduce swelling, fluid retention, and give the appearance of firmer muscle tissues. The most commonly abused drug is a diuretic, clen-buterol. Some parents hire professional scouts to secure potentially prize-winning calves for prices in excess of $15,000, and then hire professional handlers to train the animal and the youth how to manage the exhibition. When the auction price may potentially exceed $100,000, these expenses might be viewed by some parents as necessary. When the Fort Worth Stock Show first began testing champion carcasses in the 1980s, the results indi-cated that as many as half the animals had been given illegal drugs. By the mid-1990s, most livestock shows, even at the level of the smallest county fair, extracted blood, urine, and other body samples from all champions with random tests taken from other entries.

Critics contend that the increasing sale prices corrupted the educational value of the local competitions that youth exhibitions were originally in-tended to fulfill. By the mid-2000s, most state-level 4-H cooperative exten-sion offices adopted new strategies for emphasizing the value of following exhibition rules and the importance of ethical standards. Some venues, including the Houston Stock Show, have imposed a cap on the amount of cash winnings. In 2005, the grand champion steer sold for $340,000 but the exhibitor was only allowed to take home $85,000 with the rest being applied to scholarships.

Some observers, like Charles Yesalis, might link the increase in animal doping for exhibition with similar increases in anabolic steroid use among high school teens. The same parental pressures (and collusion) that emerge from such intense competition and exaggerated financial rewards are very similar to the kinds of forces that pressure teen athletes to seek chemical shortcuts through the use of anabolic steroids. The modern culture promotes external rewards as a final measure for success rather than the less obvious values of a healthy educational experience and moral character development. Yesalis would argue that the only solution to both problems is for society to reassess its cultural priorities.

CONCLUSION

"America has become a nation of *performance enhancers*" claimed an article titled, "Cheat This, Not That: Hypocrisy, Ethics and Performance Enhancement." The four coauthors had published similar articles in academic journals and were practicing professionals: one was a lawyer, another, a medical doctor, one a psychiatrist, and the last a university professor. They posted their article on a news blog hosted by an online pharmacy that sold anabolic steroids, hGH, peptides, antiestrogens, antiprolactins, and other chemical treatments for weight loss, hair loss, and erectile dysfunction, all without the need of a prescription. The article left no doubt about the authors' position on anabolic steroids—they believed that they were no different than any other medical innovation used to treat deficiencies and improve mental and physical performance. The average consumer is exposed to hundreds of hours of commercials advertising legal chemical remedies for every minor or major social ailment, from acne to baldness, from penile and breast enhancements to erectile dysfunction. Legally advertised herbal remedies promise to improve memory, mood, and concentration. Yet, anabolic steroids are isolated as a dangerous drug because they enhance performance in competitive sports. The authors argued that the primary reason behind legal sanctions and other prohibitions against ergogenic drugs was not based on clinical evidence of health risk but was instead the result of a media and academic bias that treated "those who use physique-enhancing drugs as . . . cheating, narcissistic pariahs."

A common complaint among those who oppose legal prohibitions for anabolic steroids and other ergogenic drugs is that the condemnation of such drugs reflects a moral crusade and not a medical need. As another article on the same forum explained, "The anti-doping warriors are primarily concerned with enforcing a moral code . . . [and] is not motivated to understand the true short-term and long-term health risks of anabolic steroids and performance-enhancing drugs." In fact, the advocates for strong anti-doping regulations would likely agree to part of that accusation. Yesalis, one of the most notable anti-doping crusaders, routinely called for a change in moral values as the only solution to solving the anabolic steroid epidemic. He also agreed that the mixed messages that promise instant gratification through chemical solutions greatly undermines the educational efforts of promoting a drug-free lifestyle. On this point, the two sides of the debate are in agreement—though for altogether different reasons.

Yesalis and most other such crusaders (including William Taylor, Gary Wadler, Brian Hainline, and others) would strongly disagree with the contention that they do not carefully examine the short- and long-term risks of ergogenic drugs because most of their professional work has been devoted to precisely that type of scholarly research. Nevertheless, spokespersons on both sides of the debate would agree that the real conflict is over the long-term consequences of cultural priorities rather than immediate health risks. Though individual safety and an equal playing field are the most commonly stated justifications behind the anti-doping policies of professional and amateur associations, perhaps the more influential motivation is the desire to be on the right side of the moral argument—to send the proper messages to the next generation of youth about the importance of moral character and such intrinsic values as honesty, perseverance, and individual restraint.

One of the primary roles of professional and amateur associations is to more effectively organize public opinion around a common set of values. The official policies may not be perfectly adhered to by members, but they still represent the ideal standard by which all members are held accountable. Throughout its history, the Olympic movement has struggled with athletes who use one form of ergogenic tool or another and the effort to enforce existing anti-doping rules occupies a significant percentage of the IOC resources. Yet, there is no question about the movement's official position on doping and its effect on the physical, psychological, and moral health of competing athletes. The same can be said of other professional and academic associations. The strategy of combining drug testing with broad education efforts illustrates the primary role of these associations.

One of the difficulties facing modern discussions over anabolic steroids is that the moral differences are often not explicitly addressed. Both sides of the argument agree that the anti-doping movement is promoting a particular moral position. The consensus behind most association's anti-doping rules is that ergogenic tools violate the spirit of competitive sport. That spirit usually reflects a deeper presumption about the society's moral priorities—one that holds victory is not an end in itself and it is not as important as an individual's physical, psychological, and moral well-being. The fact that a minority of voices reject that moral position demonstrates that the national consensus is not absolute, and the public debate is not over. As long as there are dissenting associations that reject that moral positions (such as the online pharmacies that sell ergogenic drugs without a prescription and advocate legalization), then the enforcement of existing laws will face some resistance.

Moral explanations can be hard to present in modern pluralist society, but pragmatic explanations that rely on public safety and an equal playing field are hard to justify without the accompanying moral reasoning. It is not surprising that the "Cheat This, Not That" article concluded with a commentary on the trend toward legalization of marijuana as a template for similar movements to legalize anabolic steroids for ergogenic use. Arguments made for or against the legalization of recreational marijuana also reflect strong presumptions about the relative importance of individual moral restraint as an intrinsic good. Immediate physical health risks of marijuana use are difficult to quantify and the primary evidence of destructive lifestyle choices rely on presumptions about what a positive lifestyle should look like.

If the spokespersons in public discussions do not include moral reasoning in their respective arguments, then the distinction between a good and a bad choice is lost. A pluralistic society may not share a strong consensus on these issues, but no legal prohibition can be sustained without clearly defining the importance of each choice. Public debate over anabolic steroids has not yet reached the level of open discussion as that of marijuana, but in the 1980s the efforts to legalize marijuana were also relegated to minority voices outside the mainstream of public debate. The distinction between use and abuse of both catabolic and anabolic steroids rests on whether they serve a therapeutic or ergogenic purposes. The relative assessments of such purposes will likely change according to the public definition of good and bad decision making. As such, the issues and controversies associated with both the therapeutic and ergogenic use of steroids will remain a lively source of public debate.

SECTION III

Primary Documents

Scientific Accounts of Anabolic and Catabolic Steroids

EXCERPT FROM C. E. BROWN-SEQUARD, *THE ELIXIR OF LIFE*

Boston: J. G. Cupples Company, 1889.

This narrative account from Dr. Brown-Sequard may well be the first clinical experimentation with anabolic steroids. The results of his tests are quite similar to what modern scientists would expect from certain anabolic steroids. Though the preparation of the elixir may cause pause for modern scientists, the prospect that some amount of testosterone was collected from the mixture is not impossible. Brown-Sequard died five years after this publication.

The Effects Produced on Man by Subcutaneous Injections of a Liquid Obtained From the Testicles of Animals

There is no need of describing at length the great effects produced on the organization of man by castration, when it is made before the adult age. It is particularly well known that eunuchs are characterized by their general debility and their lack of intellectual and physical activity. There is no medical man who does not know also how much the mind and body of men (especially before the spermatic glands have acquired their full power, or when that power is declining in consequence of advanced age) are affected by sexual abuse or by masturbation. Besides, it is well known that seminal losses, arising from any cause, produce a mental and physical debility which is in proportion to their frequency. These facts, and many others, have led to the generally-admitted view that in the seminal fluid, as secreted by the testicles, a substance or several substances exist which, entering the blood by resorption, have a most essential use in giving strength to the nervous system and to other parts. But if what may be called spermatic anemia leads to that conclusion, the opposite state, which can be named spermatic plethora, gives as strong a testimony in favor of that conclusion. It is known that well-organized men, especially from twenty to thirty-five years of age, who remain absolutely free from sexual intercourse or any other causes of expenditure of seminal fluid, are in a state of excitement, giving them a great, although abnormal, physical and mental activity. These two series of facts contribute to show what great dynamo-genie power is possessed by some substance or substances which our blood owes to the testicles.

For a great many years I have believed that the weakness of old men depended on two causes: a natural series of organic changes and the gradually diminishing action of the spermatic glands. In 1869, in a course of lectures at the Paris Faculty of Medicine, discussing the influence possessed by several glands upon the nervous centers, I put forward the idea that if it were possible without danger to inject semen into the blood of old men, we should probably obtain manifestations of increased activity as regards the mental and the various physical powers. Led by this view, I made various experiments on animals at Nahant, near Boston (United States), in 1875. In some of those experiments, made on a dozen male dogs, I tried vainly, except in one case, to engraft certain parts or the whole body of young guinea-pigs.

The success obtained in the exceptional case served to give me great hopes that by a less difficult process I should some day reach my aim. This I have now done. At the end of last year I made on two old male rabbits experiments which were repeated since on several others, with results leaving no doubt as regards both the innocuity of the process used and the good effects produced in all those animals.

This having been ascertained, I resolved to make experiments on myself, which I thought would be far more decisive on man than on animals. The event has proved the correctness of that idea. This innocuity was also proved on a very old dog by twenty subcutaneous injections of a fluid similar to that I intended to employ on myself.

No apparent harm resulted from these trials, which were made by my assistant, Dr. D' Arsonval.

For reasons I have given in many lectures in 1869 and since, I consider the spermatic as also the principal glands (kidneys, liver, etc.) as endowed, besides their secretory power, with an influence over the composition of blood, such as is possessed by the spleen, the thyroid, etc. Led by that view I have already made some trials with the blood returning from the testicles. But what I have seen is not sufficiently decisive to be mentioned here.

Leaving aside and for future researches the questions relating to the substance or substances which, being formed by the testicles, give power to the nervous centers and various other parts, I have made use, in subcutaneous injections, of a liquid containing a very small quantity of water mixed with the three following parts:

First, blood of the testicular veins;
secondly, semen; and
thirdly, juice extracted from a testicle, crushed immediately after it has been taken from a dog or a guinea-pig.

Wishing in all the injections made on myself to obtain the maximum of effects, I have employed as little water as I could. To the three kinds of substances I have just named I added distilled water in a quantity which never exceeded three or four times their volume. The crushing was always done after the addition of water. When filtered through a paper filter the liquid was of a reddish hue, and rather opaque, while it was almost perfectly clear and transparent when Pasteur's filter was employed. For each injection I have used nearly one cubic centimeter of the filtered liquid.

The animals employed were a strong, and according to all appearances, perfectly healthy dog (from two to three years old), and a number of very young or adult guinea-pigs. The experiments, so far, do not allow of a positive conclusion as regards the relative power of the liquid obtained from a dog and that drawn from guinea-pigs. All I can assert is that the two kinds of animals have given a liquid endowed with very great power. I have hitherto made ten subcutaneous injections of such a liquid—two in my left arm, all the others in my lower limbs—from May 5th to June 4th last. The first five injections were made on three succeeding days with a liquid obtained from a dog. In all the subsequent injections, made on May 24th, 29th, and 30th, and June 4th, the liquid used came from guinea-pigs. When I employed liquids having passed through Pasteur's filter, the pains and other bad effects were somewhat less than when a paper filter was used.

Coming now to the favorable effects of these injections, I beg to be excused for speaking so much as I shall do of my own person. I hope it will easily be understood, that if my demonstration has any value—I will even say any significance—it is owing to the details concerning the state of my health, strength, and habits previously to my experiments, and to the effects they have produced.

I am seventy-two years old. My general strength, which has been considerable, has notably and gradually diminished during the last ten or twelve years, Before May 15th last I was so weak that I was always compelled to sit down after an hour's work in the laboratory—even when I remained seated all the time, or almost all the time, in the laboratory, I used to come out of it quite exhausted after three or four hours' experimental labor, and sometimes after only two hours. For many years, on returning home in a carriage by six o'clock, after several hours passed in the laboratory, I was so extremely tired that I invariably had to go to bed after having hastily taken a very small amount of food. Very frequently the exhaustion was so great, that although extremely sleepy, I could not for hours go to sleep, and I only slept very little, waking up exceedingly tired.

I ought to say, that notwithstanding that dark picture, my general health is and has been almost always good, and that I had very little to complain of, excepting merycism and muscular rheumatism.

The day after the first subcutaneous injection and still more after the two succeeding ones a radical change took place in me, and I had ample reason to say and to write that I had regained at least all the strength I possessed a good many years ago. Considerable laboratory work hardly tired me. To the great astonishment of my two principal assistants, Drs. D'Arsonval and Henocque, and other persons, I was able to make experiments for several hours while standing up, feeling no need whatever to sit down. Still more: one day (the 23d of May), after three hours and a quarter of hard experimental labor in the standing attitude, I went home so little tired that after dinner I was able to go to work and to write for an hour and a half a part of a paper on a difficult subject.

For more than twenty years I had never been able to do as much. My friends know, that owing to certain circumstances and certain habits, I have for thirty or forty years gone to bed very early and done my writing work in the morning, beginning it generally between three and four o'clock. For a great many years I had lost all power of doing any serious mental work after dinner. Since my first subcutaneous injections I have very frequently been able to do such work two, three, and one evening for nearly four hours. From a natural impetuosity, and also to avoid losing time, I had, till I was sixty years old, the habit of ascending and descending stairs so rapidly that my movements were rather those of running than of walking. This had gradually changed, and I had come to move slowly up and down stairs, having to hold the banister in difficult staircases. After the second injection I found that I had fully regained my old powers, and returned to my previous habits in that respect.

My limbs, tested with a dynamometer, for a week before my trial and during the month following the first injection, showed a decided gain of strength. The average number of kilograms moved by the flexors of the right forearm, before the first injection, was about 34 1–2 (from 32 to 37), and after that injection 41 (from 39 to 44), the gain being from 6 to 7 kilograms. In that respect the fore-arm flexors reacquired, in a great measure, the strength they had when I was living in London (more than twenty-six years ago). The average number of kilograms moved by those muscles in London in 1863 was 43 (40 to 46 kilograms). I have a record of the strength of my fore-arm, begun in March, 1860, when I first established myself in London. From that time until 1862, I occasionally moved as much as fifty kilograms. During the last three years the maximum moved was thirty-eight kilograms. This year, previously to the first injection, the maximum was thirty-seven kilograms. Since the injection it has been forty-four.

I have measured comparatively, before and after the first injection, the jet of urine in similar circumstances—that is, after a meal in which I had taken food and drink of the same kind in similar quantity. The average length of the jet during the ten days that preceded the first injection was inferior by at least one quarter of what it came to be during the twenty following days. It is therefore quite evident that the power of the spinal cord over the bladder was considerably increased.

One of the most troublesome miseries of advanced life consists in the diminution of the power of defecation. To avoid repeating the details I have elsewhere given in that respect, I will simply say that after the first days of my experiments I have had a greater improvement with regard to the expulsion of fecal matters than in any other function. In fact a radical change took place, and even on days of great constipation the power I long ago possessed had returned.

With regard to the facility of intellectual labor, which had diminished within the last few years, a return to my previous ordinary condition became quite manifest during and after the first two or three days of my experiments.

It is evident from these facts and from some others that all the functions depending on the power of action of the nervous centers, and especially of the spinal cord, were notably and rapidly improved by the injections I have used. The last of these injections was made on June 4th, about five weeks and a half ago. I ceased making use of them for the purpose of ascertaining how long their good effects would last. For four weeks no marked change occurred, but gradually, although rapidly, from the 3rd of this month (July) I have witnessed almost a complete return of the state of weakness which existed before the first injection. This loss of strength is an excellent counterproof as regards the demonstration of the influence exerted on me by the subcutaneous injections of a spermatic fluid.

My first communication to the Paris Biological Society was made with the wish that other medical men advanced in life would make on themselves experiments similar to mine, so as to ascertain, as I then stated, if the effects I had observed depended or not on any special idiosyncrasy or on a kind of auto-suggestion without hypnotization, due to the conviction which I had before experimenting that I should surely obtain a great part at least of these effects. This last supposition found some ground in many of the facts contained in the valuable and learned work of Dr. Hack Tuke on the *Influence of the Mind over the Body*.

Ready as I was to make on my own person experiments which, if they were not dangerous, were at least exceedingly painful, I refused absolutely to yield to the wishes of many people anxious to obtain the effects I had observed on myself. But, without asking my advice, Dr. Variot, a physician who believed that the subcutaneous injections of considerably diluted spermatic fluid could do no harm, has made a trial of that method on three old men—one fifty-four, another fifty-six, and the third sixty-eight years old. On each of them the effects have been found to be very nearly the same as those I have obtained on myself. Dr. Variot made use of the testicles of rabbits and guinea pigs.

ADOLF WINDAUS, "CONSTITUTION OF STEROLS AND THEIR CONNECTION WITH OTHER SUBSTANCES OCCURRING IN NATURE"

Nobel Lecture, December 12, 1928. © The Nobel Foundation 1928. Used by permission.

Adolf Windaus received a Nobel Prize for Chemistry for the research he and Heinrich Wieland conducted a year earlier when they discovered the molecular structure of cholesterol. At this time, they had not yet uncovered the common relationship between cholesterol and all other steroid hormones. In this speech, Windaus suggests the possibility of hormone manipulation as a therapeutic option.

The exceptional distinction which the Royal Academy of Sciences has accorded to my work "on the sterols and their relationship to other natural products" places upon me the honour and duty of giving an account of my research to this assembly.

The sterols are nitrogen-free secondary alcohols of high molecular weight which contain in their molecules a number of alicyclic systems. A sharp distinction between the sterols and other naturally occurring hydroaromatic alcohols is not always possible.

The sterols are widely distributed in the animal, vegetable, and fungal kingdoms. The best-known sterolis cholesterol, which was first discovered in human gall-stones, and received the name cholesterol because of its presence in bile. It is a mono-unsaturated alcohol, with the formula $C_{27}H_{46}O$, found in all the higher animals, partly as free alcohol, and partly as fatty acid esters; it is present in particularly large quantities in the brain and the adrenal cortex and as a pathological deposit in gall-stones, sclerotic aorta, and other organs affected by fatty degeneration. The fluctuations of cholesterol content to which human blood serum is subject are very surprising; during pregnancy the quantity is considerably increased, while during most infectious diseases it is noticeably reduced.

In the lower animals, the insects, the echinodermata, and the sponges a number of sterols occur which are collectively known, together with cholesterol, as *zoosterols*. The majority have the same formula as cholesterol and are very similar to it; only the spongosterol, discovered by Henze in *Suberites domunculu*, appears not to be an unsaturated compound, and is more clearly differentiated from cholesterol than the other zoosterols.

In the vegetable kingdom, too, wherever they have been sought, sterols have always been found. They are grouped together as phytosterols and occur in plants partly as free alcohols and partly as glucosides. The most widely distributed are phytosterols (sitosterols) which have the same formula as cholesterol; there are, however, also phytosterols which contain not one, but two double bonds, and saturated phytosterols are also frequently mixed in small quantities with unsaturated ones. Somewhat apart from the typical sterols are sterol-like alcohols, which are differentiated from sitosterols by the number of carbon atoms, and, finally, those which contain more than one hydroxyl group. The variety of the phytosterols is therefore great, and it is noticable that, despite this great variety, animal cholesterol has never been discovered among the numerous plant sterols.

Specific sterols are also found in fungi and are classified as mycosterols. Ergosterol was first isolated from ergot by Tanret, and it is also found in numerous other fungi and especially in yeast. It has the formula $Ca_{27}H_{42}O$ and contains, in contrast to cholesterol and sitosterol, not merely one, but three double bonds. It is particularly significant that this ergosterol is mixed in very small quantities (about 1/10%) with all zoosterols and phytosterols. In addition to ergosterol still other sterols are found in fungi—zymosterol in yeast, and fungisterol in ergot. There are certainly many more.

It is surprising that in bacteria, as far as they have been examined, no sterols occur. Panzer noted their absence from tuberculous and diphtheria bacilli, and

I can confirm this result for the tubercule bacilli, as I have worked on several kilogrammes of these. I have shown by physiological means that ergosterol does not occur even in traces in tubercle wax.

Chemically by far the most thoroughly examined is the sterol of the higher animals, cholesterol. The laborious and protracted investigation of its constitution has shown that it probably possesses the structure (I). According to Wieland's research this formula may be resolved into the complete structural formula (II). This formula is very complicated and has no similarity to the formulae of sugar, fatty acids, or the amino acids which occur in protein.

The synthesis of such a substance appears to the chemist particularly difficult, and up till now I have not dared to attempt it, as success is extremely improbable. Furthermore, the majority of physiologists have not been inclined to believe the animal organism capable of such a synthesis, for it is known that other, seemingly simpler, syntheses—e.g. that of tyrosine and tryptophan—have not succeeded in the animal organism.

If the human and animal organism were really not in a position to produce cholesterol from other constituents, then the cholesterol of the higher animals, the carnivores and herbivores, would necessarily originate in their food. But as the herbivore does not receive cholesterol but phytosterol in its food, it must possess the ability to absorb the phytosterol of its vegetable nourishment and to convert it to cholesterol.

To test this assumption Schonheimer carried out experiments on rabbits in the Institute of Pathology in Freiburg. He found 96.9% of the ingested sitosterol (0.2 g per day) in the excrement, and concluded from this that sitosterol is not absorbed by the intestinal canal of the rabbit. There can therefore be no question of the herbivore using the phytosterol in its food to form the cholesterol of its body substance. On the contrary, it must be in the position to form cholesterol from other components of its nourishment.

Whether or not mycosterols behave like phytosterols still remains to be accurately established. On the other hand, it is known that cholesterol, which is so extremely similar to sitosterol in its physical and chemical properties, behaves physiologically in quite a different manner. It is absorbed by both herbivores and carnivores and particularly easily when bile salts are available in abundance. Schonheimer found only 50% of the ingested cholesterol (0.2 g per day) in the excrement of rabbits. Furthermore, the cholesterol content of the blood is greatly increased after feeding with cholesterol, and it is noticeable that after long periods of feeding with cholesterol symptoms of disease appear in the animal. Mice, rats, and cats accumulate cholesterol, which is introduced with the food, principally in the liver, so that the cholesterol content of this organ can increase to more than five times normal, and a severe anisotropic fatty degeneration of the liver becomes apparent. If small doses of cholesterol are fed to rabbits deposits occur at first only in the intima of the blood vessel, which is the organ most sensitive to cholesterol in the rabbit. This observation is of very great interest, for according to Aschoff a disease pattern arises at this point which is identical with that of arteriosclerosis in man. The hypothesis of a genetic connection between ingested cholesterol and arteriosclerosis in man thus cannot be dismissed. Since phytosterols, which cannot be absorbed, bring about no such symptoms, it should be investigated whether or not true arteriosclerosis presents itself in societies which are truly vegetarian (abstaining also from milk and eggs).

Although the animal thus is in a position to absorb cholesterol from its food with the aid of bile salts, nevertheless not even the carnivore is dependent on this cholesterol introduced from outside. As Beumer has demonstrated, puppies fed on a diet deficient in cholesterol exhibit after four weeks an increase of cholesterol which is twenty times greater than the amount given in the food. Particularly painstaking have been the investigations of Randles and Knudson into the question of a cholesterol synthesis. They have succeeded in maintaining white rats on a diet completely free of sterols, on the basis of the discovery that pulverized alfalfa, on extraction with cold ether, relinquishes its sterols completely, but retains enough vitamins for the maintenance of rats. The scientists mentioned reached the incontestable conclusion that the cholesterol content of fully-grown rats fed on a diet free of cholesterol is many times greater than the cholesterol content of new-born rats. The only possible explanation for this is that the organism of the rat is capable of forming cholesterol from substances which are different from the sterols and other substances soluble in ether.

There is thus in the animal organism a cholesterol synthesis, and the synthetic capabilities of the animal have been gravely underestimated here, as in many other cases.

PAUL DE KRUIF, *THE MALE HORMONE*

New York: Harcourt, Brace and Company, 1945, pp. 3, 7–8, 35, 101, 108, 120–123, 139, 198, 224, 226.

This excerpt is intended to show the state of knowledge of steroids when they were first being researched. The emphasis and motivation was primarily as an antiaging solution. It was not researched as an ergogenic drug, so most observers did not automatically associate testosterone with cheating in sports. It was another 20 years or more before people began to see these chemical supplements as primarily ergogenic in nature and potentially dangerous. It is that later association that prompted the birth of anti-doping policies that came later. It is important to know though that this 1945 antiaging discussion was almost entirely in terms of a therapeutic solution to age as if it were a disease. There is little to no mention of testosterone use for purely cosmetic purposes. Could it be argued that some of the current concerns about anabolic steroid use are that it is most associated with ergogenic or cosmetic use and not as a therapeutic option for general old age? Careful examination may find Kruif discussing this possibility even in 1945. Paul de Kruif died two days before his 81st birthday.

Fifteen years ago this Autumn I began writing a story about men against death that opened with the too obvious words, "I don't want to die." I was then thirty-nine years old and strong, swimming in Lake Michigan, like a slightly middle-aged walrus, vain of that strength, yet haunted by a scientific promise that it was not likely to be mine for many years longer. Warnings from the life tablets showed that, getting the breaks of the average man, there were only twenty more years to live. It was far too short. There was so much left to learn before I could attain the beginning of wisdom, so much of my past life to atone for before I could hope to become a decent man. At the same time, a great deal of study had shown me that science had already done about as much as could be expected in delaying the aging of my muscles, brain, bones and arteries.

To tell the truth, medical science had been an absolute flop in its unorganized and feeble effort to check the dissolution and death that marched toward all middle-aged men and women. Men of science cut themselves splendid pieces of cake for their saving of babies, children and young people from many microbic deaths, but they had nothing to offer to push back the on-rushing disease of old age. It seems as cruel as it was idiotic and wasteful. It seemed as if the young were preserved to a time of the beginning of wisdom and serene enjoyment of life, then to begin to crack up with the diseases of degeneration, then to be told by science, "We were only fooling you."

. . . It was Doctor Herman N. Bundesen, President of the Chicago Board of Health, who first held out to me a will-o'-wisp of hope that, though it may not be possible to throw advancing age into reverse, yet there might be a gleam of chemical promise of prolonging what was left of my prime of life. He intimated that the disintegration that scared me *might* be partly due to a hormone hunger.

Hormones? They were supposed to be the chemical messengers of the animal body. Hormones of innumerable kinds were supposed to be manufactured by various organs and glands in the body, to pass into the blood, and then to excite different and distant parts of the body to chemical activity.

I knew that insulin was one such hormone, manufactured by the pancreas, and thyroxin another typical hormone manufactured by the thyroid gland. Then too I had heard of the female hormones, estrone and estradiol, made by the ovaries. I knew that the testicles secreted testosterone (acvcent on the second syllable and rhyming with alone) but beyond this my knowledge of hormones was vague.

This was in the early nineteen-forties, and I listened skeptically to Herman Bundesen's mysterious hints about this new hormone science. I had a vague idea that his view of it wasn't exactly medically orthodox. The possibility of any restoration of man's waning energy by the male sex hormone particularly (and this was what Bundesen hinted) was certainly not generally admitted by the authorities on the new science of hormone who were discussing the subject in widely read journals. Moreover the idea sounded fishy because it was sexy—and who hadn't heard that monkey glands were the bunk? Yet, knowing Herman Bundesen as I was coming to do, I thought twice before selling him short on any medical project that he sponsored."

. . . These events of the nineteen-twenties and nineteen-thirties could be called miracles in cold scientific print. Once the organize chemists had got them absolutely pure, or even sufficiently concentrated, they unlocked doors that, from time's beginning, had been slammed shut by death. If insulin, if liver extract, if pure vitamins, could make these miracles, then maybe Bundesen might be right when he hinted at the pure male hormone's power to revive and prolong the total vitality of men . . .

Pondering the history of the male hormone I pinched myself to see if I was awake or only dreaming. It seemed too clear-cut and simple. Could it be that testosterone was going to be found to be the master key to unlock waning total vitality in men? These pre-puberty and post-puberty euchuchoids were exactly the human experimental animals that you needed to test it, precisely like laboratory castrated white rats or capons. The experimental human material was yelling to be tested. There were plenty of God-forsaken men who'd been bereft of their sex glands by war wounds, by industrial accidents, by mumps, tuberculosis, and other diseases. Now that the news of testosterone was getting about by these first publications and by the scientific grapevine, the doctors would certainly begin rounding up these unfortunates . . .

The power of testosterone was beyond the merely sexual. Many of these almost-men and broken men showed a new surge of general strength and energy; and there was a rapid increase in the muscular development of several of them. One of them who had been especially shy, bashful, and hating to associate with men of his own age, changed remarkably. He became self-confident and optimistic. All of these forlorn and formerly feeble fellows became more aggressive and quicker on the trigger andf more capable in their daily work. In every instance there was extraordinary improvement in their spirits, in what the doctors called their psychological outlook. They were hopeful now and cheerful.

The power of testosterone was more than a flash in the pan. These twenty-two men were continued under the treatment for two years, and there was no waning of their new manhood, and all of them clamored to keep on taking these life-giving injections.

There seemed no doubt that testosterone was the complete answer to a lack of the male hormone that's the internal secretion of the human testicles.

Nobody could object to this magic new life for the almost men and the resurrection of those castrates whose lives had been broken. But, looked at in the broadest moral sense, when this new testosterone got into real chemical mass production (it was still rare and expensive) wouldn't it then be dangerous, be dynamite to turn loose on humanity? After all these forlorn eunuchoids had a right to normal life, and they were no great part of humanity, in numbers. But what about testosterone's possible effect upon our young men who were already too, too sexual and wanted to be still more so? It was a disturbing question for clergymen, social workers, and all upright and serious citizens . . .

There was now a new form of the pure male hormone, methyl testosterone that you could give in the form of simple pills by mouth, far more practical than the old testosterone proprionate that had to be given in a doctor's office by injections. Ten of these pills, given daily to these broken men, quickly raised their weight-lifting power by seventy-six per cent, raised their weight-holding power by forty-one per cent; and they recovered thirty per cent faster after tiring. The testosterone pills not only increased their muscular endurance but cut down the *fatigability* of their nervous systems; you could measure that by the way their eyes increased their power to distinguish the flickering of a rapidly flashing light.

But what interested me most deeply was that this magical effect of testosterone upon the vigor of nerves and muscles *wasn't confined to eunuchoid almost-men and broken men.* It wasn't as the John Hopkins doctors had led me to believe. These Milwaukee biological engineers made determinations of testosterone's action on men with testicles, men from fifty-three to sixty-seven years old, who'd come simply complaining of various nervous symptoms, of being very, very tired from very little work; and they were impotent.

While the response to testosterone was far less striking than it had been in those eunuchoids, yet aging men, too, showed a definite, measurable improvement in the power of their nerves and muscles . . .

The effect of the pure male hormone on a normal, sexually competent young man, thirty-seven years old, was curious. An injection of testosterone did not make him sexually more so. In fact, its effect was opposite; it definitely lowered his sex desire and drive. But at the same time his muscular tone and his endurance went up, definitely.

It was clear that testosterone did not turn a young man into a Don Juan, yet it might have a definite up-surging effect on his total vitality . . . [Dr. Walter Kearns] warned against the misuse of testosterone now that you could take it in the form of pills, and now that its increasing production was beginning to make it cheaper . . .

Rejuvenation's no dirty word to anybody clearly understanding testosterone's action. "Successful rejuvenation for the aged," Kearns said, "brings about clearer mental processes, better functions of the vital organs, a marked increase in energy and drive and a decided uplift in mental outlook."

. . . "That rejuvenation *may* bring with it a return of sexual activity is of secondary importance," he said . . .

I'll never forget the day he gave me those first tablets, little ten milligram pills not much bigger than an asperin, for my own use . . . Now I'd been on them a year, faithfully; and it seemed as if there was a bit of an up in my spirits, a bit more optimism, maybe . . ."

I will try to renew my aging tissues with testosterone as long as I can . . . And what if testosterone, raising my total vitality, making me burn the candle at both ends, does make me die sooner? I'd rather live not so long, but with my total vitality on a high sprocket, than drag along at a lower level of living, saving myself till I'd pass out at last, a drooling dotard at ninety. It's only a little longer prime of life I'm after.

So I'll try fortifying my aging tissues according to the prescription of Herman Bundesen, according to his hunch that the male hormone may super-charge them just as chemicals renew worn-out soil . . .

Now I'm fifty-four years old, and there's so much left to do. I've grown old much too quick and smart much too late, but at least I'm this much wiser than fifteen years ago, when I was sobbing a but about not wanting to die . . .

Now I see a gleam of hope of science to help me extend the prime of my life. I do not say it is more than a glimmer. I feel that testosterone has already helped me. Of course the male hormone isn't the whole story. I'll watch my nutrition and go on supercharging myself with vitamins just to be on the safe side . . .

So, no different than a good diabetic child who knows that insulin every day makes the difference between living and dying, I'll be faithful and remember to take my twenty or thirty milligrams a day of testosterone. I'm not ashamed that it's no longer made to its old degree by my own aging body. It's chemical crutches. It's borrowed manhood. It's borrowed time. But, just the same, it's what makes bulls bulls. And, who knows, maybe tomorrow, they'll hit on a simple dietary chemical trick that will, to a degree, bring back the power of the glands that make my own natural male hormone.

APPENDIX B

Documents Related to Legal Sanctions

The government reacted to the rising chemical culture of the 1960s by creating a uniform system of classifying and controlling drugs according to their therapeutic value as balanced against their potential for addiction. The first of these documents provides the justification for the initial classification system, and includes specific provisions for adding new designations and revising existing ones. Based on the existing law, what would justify possible future legalization of anabolic steroids for nontherapeutic use? The second of these documents is from a Senate Hearing investigating the role of steroids in amateur sports. What threats did anabolic steroids use pose to society as cited by the lawmaker?

CONTROLLED SUBSTANCES ACT

U.S. Code, Title 21, Chapter 13. Sections 801, 801a, 811, and 812.

TITLE 21—FOOD AND DRUGS
CHAPTER 13—DRUG ABUSE PREVENTION AND CONTROL
SUBCHAPTER I—CONTROL AND ENFORCEMENT

§ 801. Congressional Findings and Declarations: Controlled Substances

The Congress makes the following findings and declarations:

(1) Many of the drugs included within this subchapter have a useful and legitimate medical purpose and are necessary to maintain the health and general welfare of the American people.
(2) The illegal importation, manufacture, distribution, and possession and improper use of controlled substances have a substantial and detrimental effect on the health and general welfare of the American people. . .

(6) Federal control of the intrastate incidents of the traffic in controlled substances is essential to the effective control of the interstate incidents of such traffic.

(7) The United States is a party to the Single Convention on Narcotic Drugs, 1961, and other international conventions designed to establish effective control over international and domestic traffic in controlled substances.

§ 801a. Congressional Findings and Declarations: Psychotropic Substances

The Congress makes the following findings and declarations:

(1) The Congress has long recognized the danger involved in the manufacture, distribution, and use of certain psychotropic substances for nonscientific and nonmedical purposes, and has provided strong and effective legislation to control illicit trafficking and to regulate legitimate uses of psychotropic substances in this country. Abuse of psychotropic substances has become a phenomenon common to many countries, however, and is not confined to national borders. It is, therefore, essential that the United States cooperate with other nations in establishing effective controls over international traffic in such substances. . .

(3) In implementing the Convention on Psychotropic Substances, the Congress intends that, consistent with the obligations of the United States under the Convention, control of psychotropic substances in the United States should be accomplished within the framework of the procedures and criteria for classification of substances provided in the Comprehensive Drug Abuse Prevention and Control Act of 1970 (21 U.S.C. 801 et seq.). This will insure that

(A) the availability of psychotropic substances to manufacturers, distributors, dispensers, and researchers for useful and legitimate medical and scientific purposes will not be unduly restricted;

(B) nothing in the Convention will interfere with bona fide research activities; and

(C) nothing in the Convention will interfere with ethical medical practice in this country as determined by the Secretary of Health and Human Services on the basis of a consensus of the views of the American medical and scientific community. . .

(41)

(A) The term "anabolic steroid" means any drug or hormonal substance, chemically and pharmacologically related to testosterone (other than estrogens, progestins, and corticosteroids) that promotes muscle growth, and includes. . .

(B)

(i) Except as provided in clause (ii), such term does not include an anabolic steroid which is expressly intended for administration through implants to cattle or other nonhuman species and which has been approved by the Secretary of Health and Human Services for such administration.

(ii) If any person prescribes, dispenses, or distributes such steroid for human use, such person shall be considered to have prescribed, dispensed, or distributed an anabolic steroid within the meaning of subparagraph (A). . .

PART B—AUTHORITY TO CONTROL; STANDARDS AND SCHEDULES

§ 811. Authority and Criteria for Classification of Substances. . .

(c) Factors determinative of control or removal from schedules

In making any finding under subsection (a) of this section or under subsection (b) of section 812 of this title, the Attorney General shall consider the following factors with respect to each drug or other substance proposed to be controlled or removed from the schedules:

(1) Its actual or relative potential for abuse.
(2) Scientific evidence of its pharmacological effect, if known.
(3) The state of current scientific knowledge regarding the drug or other substance.
(4) Its history and current pattern of abuse.
(5) The scope, duration, and significance of abuse.
(6) What, if any, risk there is to the public health.
(7) Its psychic or physiological dependence liability.
(8) Whether the substance is an immediate precursor of a substance already controlled under this subchapter. . .

§ 812. Schedules of Controlled Substances

(a)   Establishment

There are established five schedules of controlled substances, to be known as schedules I, II, III, IV, and V. Such schedules shall initially consist of the substances listed in this section. The schedules established by this section shall be updated and republished on a semiannual basis during the two-year period beginning one year after October 27, 1970, and shall be updated and republished on an annual basis thereafter.

(b)   Placement on schedules; findings required

Except where control is required by United States obligations under an international treaty, convention, or protocol, in effect on October 27, 1970, and except in the case of an immediate precursor, a drug or other substance may not be placed in any schedule unless the findings required for such schedule are made with respect to such drug or other substance. The findings required for each of the schedules are as follows:

(1) Schedule I.-

    (A) The drug or other substance has a high potential for abuse.

    (B) The drug or other substance has no currently accepted medical use in treatment in the United States.

    (C) There is a lack of accepted safety for use of the drug or other substance under medical supervision.

(2) Schedule II.-

    (A) The drug or other substance has a high potential for abuse.

    (B) The drug or other substance has a currently accepted medical use in treatment in the United States or a currently accepted medical use with severe restrictions.

    (C) Abuse of the drug or other substances may lead to severe psychological or physical dependence.

(3) Schedule III.-

    (A) The drug or other substance has a potential for abuse less than the drugs or other substances in schedules I and II.

    (B) The drug or other substance has a currently accepted medical use in treatment in the United States.

    (C) Abuse of the drug or other substance may lead to moderate or low physical dependence or high psychological dependence.

(4) Schedule IV.-

    (A) The drug or other substance has a low potential for abuse relative to the drugs or other substances in schedule III.

    (B) The drug or other substance has a currently accepted medical use in treatment in the United States.

    (C) Abuse of the drug or other substance may lead to limited physical dependence or psychological dependence relative to the drugs or other substances in schedule III.

(5) Schedule V.-

    (A) The drug or other substance has a low potential for abuse relative to the drugs or other substances in schedule IV.

    (B) The drug or other substance has a currently accepted medical use in treatment in the United States.

    (C) Abuse of the drug or other substance may lead to limited physical dependence or psychological dependence relative to the drugs or other substances in schedule IV. . .

§ 814. Removal of Exemption of Certain Drugs

    (a) Removal of exemption

The Attorney General shall by regulation remove from exemption under section 802(39)(A)(iv) of this title a drug or group of drugs that the Attorney General finds is being diverted to obtain a listed chemical for use in the illicit production of a controlled substance.

(b)   Factors to be considered

In removing a drug or group of drugs from exemption under subsection (a) of this section, the Attorney General shall consider, with respect to a drug or group of drugs that is proposed to be removed from exemption-

   (1)   the scope, duration, and significance of the diversion;
   (2)   whether the drug or group of drugs is formulated in such a way that it cannot be easily used in the illicit production of a controlled substance; and
   (3)   whether the listed chemical can be readily recovered from the drug or group of drugs.

ABUSE OF ANABOLIC STEROIDS AND THEIR PRECURSORS BY ADOLESCENT AMATEUR ATHLETES

TUESDAY, JULY 13, 2004
United States Senate, Caucus on International Narcotics Control, Washington, DC.
The Caucus met, pursuant to notice, at 9:52 a.m., in room SD-215, Dirksen Senate Office Building, Hon. Charles E. Grassley, Chairman of the Caucus, presiding.
Present: Senators Grassley and Biden.

Opening Statement of Hon. Charles E. Grassley, U.S. Senator from IOWA

Chairman Grassley. Good morning, everybody, and I appreciate everybody who has come, and we are getting started just a little bit early. Normally I do not start without a member of the minority present, but Senator Biden is the Vice Chairman here, and he commutes regularly. His train is a little bit late, but he gave permission for us to go ahead, so I am going to start.

For more than two decades, the use of steroids by professional athletes has been widely reported. Indictments against executive officers of a San Francisco area nutritional supplements lab—and these indictments were Federal steroid distribution charges—have brought even more attention to the use of steroids. Recently, accusations of world-class track and baseball athletes using steroids have hit the news. But steroid use often begins even before athletes achieve international recognition.

Today's hearing will focus on the availability of illegal steroids and, of course, on the pressures that young athletes face to use steroids to improve their performance. Anabolic steroids are easily purchased over the Internet, as well as from users who sell and distribute steroids in gyms. The ease with which anybody, including young people, can acquire these drugs, coupled with the high percentage of purchased steroids that are counterfeit, even heighten the severe health risks to the users.

Recent studies have shown that the use of illegal steroids has skyrocketed among high-school and college athletes. Despite the widely publicized danger of anabolic steroid abuse, it is estimated that as many as 5 million people annually, even including 175,000 high-school girls and 350,000 high-school-aged boys, may be abusing these drugs to improve athletic performance, appearance, and self-image. In fact, those same studies have shown that some users start even younger, first using steroids while they are in middle-school. These children are taking drugs to gain immediate enhancement of athletic performance.

What has been most troubling is that some coaches, the very people we entrust to teach fair sportsmanship to our children and to care for their well-being, are promoting the use of steroids. The mind-set that winning comes before all else says to our kids that they should do whatever it takes to get bigger, to get stronger, and to get faster. Too often, young athletes see steroid use as the only way to comply with that coach's demand. Winning at all costs places too great a risk to the health of our children and undermines the element of fairness that we expect in sporting competition.

When I started to look at this problem, I was amazed at just how easy it is to get this poison. I found several websites where steroids and precursors can be purchased online.

In fact, I found illegal steroids available on eBay! And if that is not bad enough, young athletes can buy the needles used to inject the illegal steroids directly into their bodies on eBay as well.

Example 1 that I show you here shows one of these sales on eBay where they advertise 1-inch needles to inject, and I quote, "DECA, D-BOL, TEST." These are all terms for illegal steroids. This web page also says that these needles, and I quote, are "a must for those with gear," and the word "gear" being a common code word for steroids.

A second example, also taken from eBay, shows just how easy it is to buy steroids. Now, notice the category at the top of the poster that says the drugs are listed under "Health and Beauty." Quite ironic, actually. We will hear from one witness, Dr. Catlin, a leading expert on steroids, about the clear dangers to the health of those who take these illegal drugs. We will also hear from Don Hooten, whose son, Taylor, committed suicide as a result of abusing illegal steroids. Now, when you get right down to it, what beauty is there in the death of a young student?

Again, example 2 offers the illegal steroid D-bol or Dianabol to any willing bidder. This fellow says that D-bol pills he is selling are, and I quote, "the real deal" and that he "used them personally and they're awesome." A personal endorsement, and according to this example, you get free shipping to boot!

We have example 3 that shows how easy it is to get injectable steroids on the Internet. This seller has 10 ampules of Sustanon and 10 ampules of Deca-Durabolin. That's referred to as "Deca." This seller tries to pretend that he does not know what these drugs will be used for when he says, and I quote, "For vet use only." What veterinarian would buy his medications on eBay?

Injectable steroids are particularly dangerous to young abusers who do not know how to inject needles correctly. Infections, nerve damage, and even deadly disease can occur from the use of needles. Injecting steroids directly into the vein or artery can cause serious health risks.

Others use clever tricks to hide their criminal intent. In example 4, this guy claims to be selling a "picture of D-bol." Just a picture. Included in the description, he tells the buyer the lot number and expiration date of the picture. Indeed, he says, "The picture comes in a sealed container with free priority mail." By the way, the picture sold for $60.

In example 5, we see a seller who advertises a list of steroid distributors that he got from "steroidworld.com." The seller says that he has "100 percent success rate" and that the sellers on the list will, and I quote, "use labels which will hide the package's contents."

So, I hope it is quite obvious and clear that these products are readily available. But to make matters worse, counterfeit steroids are also being sold widely. These fake drugs are very convincing in appearance. In front of us, you can see several examples of high-quality counterfeit steroids. Notice the quality of the packaging, labeling, and inserts that are on the table. These steroids are fake but convincing. We will hear more about this today from a former steroid distributor and user, who will testify that 95 percent of the steroids on the market are not genuine. Fake steroids have been known to have a mixture of cooking oil—can you believe this?—even motor oil in the package. Imagine a high-school student injecting motor oil into his or her body.

I hope that today's witnesses will help us all understand the problems here as well as some of the efforts being made to confront this menace. In addition to the testimony that we will hear today, we have also received written testimony from several different groups, which, if there is no objection, I will include in the record.

Anti-Doping Policies from Associations

These documents illustrate the milestones in the history of anti-doping policies as instituted through sports associations. As international bodies, the only legal authority these associations have is the suspension, prohibition, or elimination of an athlete's ability to participate in their organized events. As samples of historical change over time, how do these documents reflect the changing view of ergogenic drugs? Which concerns receive the greatest priority: fair play, athletic safety, or integrity of the sport? Do these priorities change over time? How do these associations distinguish between therapeutic and ergogenic use?

INTERNATIONAL AMATEUR ATHLETIC FEDERATION

Handbook of the International Amateur Athletic Federation, 1927–1928, IAAF: Monaco, 1928, pp. 39, 55. Used by permission of the IAAF.

Section 13. >>*Doping*>> (Comp. Section 22.) [p.39]

The Council having studied the question of >>doping>> in its sessions during the Olympic Games proposed to the Congress, that a rule should be made prohibiting the use of drugs or stimulants in athletic competitions. The Congress voted unanimously that such a rule should be introduced, whereupon a lively discussion ensured as to the text to be adopted in this respect. The various propositions and amendments were handed over to the Council which was asked by the Congress to present a definite text to be adopted by the Congress at the next day's meeting . . .

Section 22. >>Doping>> (Comp. Section 13.)

According to the decision reported in Section 13 the Council had again studied the question of >>doping>> and proposed that the following rule be accepted by the Congress:

>>Doping is the use of any stimulant not normally employed to increase the power of action in athletic competition above the average.

Any person knowingly acting or assisting as explained above shall be excluded from any place where these rules are in force or, if he is a competitor, be suspended for a time or otherwise from further participation in amateur athletics under the jurisdiction of this Federation.>>

After a short discussion, the proposition of the Council was accepted.

OLYMPIC MOVEMENT MEDICAL CODE

Used by permission of the IOC Medical Commission
In force as from 1 October 2009

Preamble

"Fundamental Principles of Olympism

1. Olympism is a philosophy of life, exalting and combining in a balanced whole the qualities of body, will and mind. Blending sport with culture and education, Olympism seeks to create a way of life based on the joy of effort, the educational value of good example and respect for universal fundamental ethical principles.
2. The goal of Olympism is to place sport at the service of the harmonious development of man, with a view to promoting a peaceful society concerned with the preservation of human dignity."

Olympic Charter, July 2007

1. The Olympic Movement, in accomplishing its mission, should encourage all stakeholders to take measures to ensure that sport is practised without danger to the health of the athletes and with respect for fair play and sports ethics. To that end, it encourages those measures necessary to protect the health of participants and to minimise the risks of physical injury and psychological harm. It also encourages measures that will protect athletes in their relationships with physicians and other health care providers.
2. This objective can be achieved mainly through an ongoing education based on the ethical values of sport and on each individual's responsibility in protecting his or her health and the health of others.
3. The present Code supports the basic rules regarding best medical practices in the domain of sport and the safeguarding of the rights and health of the athletes. It supports and encourages the adoption of specific measures to achieve those objectives. It complements and reinforces the

World Anti-Doping Code as well as the general principles recognised in international codes of medical ethics.

4. The Olympic Movement Medical Code is directed toward the Olympic Games, championships of the International Federations and competitions to which the International Olympic Committee (IOC) grants its patronage or support, and to all sport practised within the context of the Olympic Movement, both during training

2012–2013 NCAA LIST OF BANNED DRUGS

Used by permission of the NCAA.

It is the student-athlete's responsibility to check with the appropriate or designated athletics staff before using any substance

The NCAA bans the following classes of drugs:

a. Stimulants
b. Anabolic Agents
c. Alcohol and Beta Blockers (banned for rifle only)
d. Diuretics and Other Masking Agents
e. Street Drugs
f. Peptide Hormones and Analogues
g. Anti-estrogens
h. Beta-2 Agonists

Note: Any substance chemically related to these classes is also banned.

The institution and the student-athlete shall be held accountable for all drugs within the banned drug class regardless of whether they have been specifically identified.

Drugs and Procedures Subject to Restrictions:

a. Blood Doping.
b. Local Anesthetics (under some conditions).
c. Manipulation of Urine Samples.
d. Beta-2 Agonists permitted only by prescription and inhalation.
e. Caffeine if concentrations in urine exceed 15 micrograms/ml.

NCAA Nutritional/Dietary Supplements Warning:

Before consuming any nutritional/dietary supplement product, review the product with the appropriate or designated athletics department staff!

- Dietary supplements are not well regulated and may cause a positive drug test result.
- Student-athletes have tested positive and lost their eligibility using dietary supplements.

- Many dietary supplements are contaminated with banned drugs not listed on the label.
- Any product containing a dietary supplement ingredient is taken at your own risk.

Note to Student-Athletes: There is no complete list of banned substances.
Do not rely on this list to rule out any supplement ingredient. Check with your athletics department staff prior to using a supplement.
Some Examples of NCAA Banned Substances in Each Drug Class

Stimulants: amphetamine (Adderall); caffeine (guarana); cocaine; ephedrine; fenfluramine (Fen); methamphetamine; methylphenidate (Ritalin); phentermine (Phen); synephrine (bitter orange); methylhexaneamine, "bath salts" (mephedrone) etc. Exceptions: phenylephrine and pseudoephedrine are not banned.

Anabolic Agents (sometimes listed as a chemical formula, such as 3,6,17-androstenetrione): boldenone; clenbuterol; DHEA (7-Keto); nandrolone; stanozolol; testosterone; methasterone; androstenedione; norandrostenedione; methandienone; etiocholanolone; trenbolone; etc.

Alcohol and Beta Blockers (banned for rifle only): alcohol; atenolol; metoprolol; nadolol; pindolol; propranolol; timolol; etc.

Diuretics (water pills) and Other Masking Agents: bumetanide; chlorothiazide; furosemide; hydrochlorothiazide; probenecid; spironolactone (canrenone); triameterene; trichlormethiazide; etc.

Street Drugs: heroin; marijuana; tetrahydrocannabinol (THC); synthetic cannabinoids (eg. spice, K2, JWH-018, JWH-073)

Peptide Hormones and Analogues: growth hormone(hGH); human chorionic gonadotropin (hCG); erythropoietin (EPO); etc.

Anti-Estrogens: anastrozole; tamoxifen; formestane; 3,17-dioxo-etiochol-1,4,6-triene(ATD), etc.

Beta-2 Agonists: bambuterol; formoterol; salbutamol; salmeterol; etc.

Any substance that is chemically related to the class, even if it is not listed as an example, is also banned!

UNIVERSITY INTERSCHOLASTIC LEAGUE (UIL) ANTI-DOPING CONTRACT

Used by permission of the University Interscholastic League.

UIL is the organization that Texas uses to test high school athletes, which has been mandated by Texas State Law.

Steroid Agreement 2013–2014

Parent and Student Agreement/
Acknowledgement Form
Anabolic Steroid Use and Random Steroid Testing

- Texas state law prohibits possessing, dispensing, delivering or administering a steroid in a manner not allowed by state law.
- Texas state law also provides that body building, muscle enhancement or the increase in muscle bulk or strength through the use of a steroid by a person who is in good health is not a valid medical purpose.
- Texas state law requires that only a licensed practitioner with prescriptive authority may prescribe a steroid for a person.
- Any violation of state law concerning steroids is a criminal offense punishable by confinement in jail or imprisonment in the Texas Department of Criminal Justice.

STUDENT ACKNOWLEDGEMENT AND AGREEMENT

As a prerequisite to participation in UIL athletic activities, I agree that I will not use anabolic steroids as defined in the UIL Anabolic Steroid Testing Program Protocol. I have read this form and understand that I may be asked to submit to testing for the presence of anabolic steroids in my body, and I do hereby agree to submit to such testing and analysis by a certified laboratory. I further understand and agree that the results of the steroid testing may be provided to certain individuals in my high school as specified in the UIL Anabolic Steroid Testing Program Protocol which is available on the UIL website at www.uiltexas.org. I understand and agree that the results of steroid testing will be held confidential to the extent required by law. I understand that failure to provide accurate and truthful information could subject me to penalties as determined by UIL.

Student Name (Print): _____ Grade (9–12) _____
Student Signature: _____ Date: _____

PARENT/GUARDIAN CERTIFICATION AND ACKNOWLEDGEMENT

As a prerequisite to participation by my student in UIL athletic activities, I certify and acknowledge that I have read this form and understand that my student must refrain from anabolic steroid use and may be asked to submit to testing for the presence of anabolic steroids in his/her body. I do hereby agree to submit my child to such testing and analysis by a certified laboratory. I further understand and agree that the results of the steroid testing may be provided to certain individuals in my student's high school as specified in the UIL Anabolic Steroid Testing Program Protocol which is available on the UIL website at www.uiltexas.org. I understand and agree that the results of steroid testing will be held confidential to the extent required by law. I understand that failure to provide accurate and truthful information could subject my student to penalties as determined by UIL.

Name (Print): _____

Signature: _____ Date: _____

Relationship to student: _____

UNIVERSITY INTERSCHOLASTIC LEAGUE (UIL) STEROIDS TESTING SITE COORDINATOR MANUAL

Used by permission of the University Interscholastic League.

This includes the excerpts related to procedures and the list of banned substances.

Procedure

At the Start of the School Year

At the beginning of each school year, UIL member schools shall identify one (1) Member School Representative (MSR) and two (2) individuals (one male and one female) to serve as Testing Site Coordinators (TSC) to assist with the crew chief assigned to that testing event.

Your school must have obtained the required acknowledgement and consent forms from each high school student-athlete as listed below.

A Student-athlete is prohibited from participating in an athletic competition sponsored or sanctioned by the UIL unless:

1) the student-athlete agrees not to use anabolic steroids; and,
2) if enrolled in high school, the student-athlete submits to random testing for the presence of anabolic steroids in the student-athlete's body; and
3) the school obtains from the student-athlete's parent, a UIL approved acknowledgement and consent form signed by the parent and acknowledging that:
   a. the parent or guardian's child, if enrolled in high school, may be subject to random anabolic steroid testing; and
   b. the parent or guardian consents to such testing; and
   c. state law prohibits possessing, dispensing, delivering, or administering a steroid in a manner not allowed by state law;
   d. state law provides that bodybuilding, muscle enhancement, or the increase of muscle bulk or strength through the use of a steroid by a person who is in good health is not a valid medical purpose;
   e. only a licensed practitioner with prescriptive authority may prescribe a steroid for a person; and
   f. a violation of state law concerning steroids is a criminal offense punishable by confinement in jail or imprisonment in the Texas Department of Criminal Justice.

The UIL Parent and Student Notification/Agreement Form for Illegal Steroid Use and Random Steroid Testing addresses all the above requirements.

When Your School is Notified of Anabolic Steroid Testing

For anabolic steroid testing events, the MSR and TSCs will be officially notified of the anabolic steroid testing event a minimum of twenty-four (24) hours (1 business day) but no more than forty-eight (48) hours (2 business days) before the day of testing by Drug Free Sport. Drug Free Sport will notify the MSR and the two TSCs by either facsimile or by email.

The MSR, TSCs and/or any other school personnel notified of an anabolic steroid testing event are required to keep such notification confidential. Failure of the MSR, TSC(s) and/or any other school personnel so notified to keep such notification information confidential will be considered a violation of UIL rules and appropriate sanctions from the range of penalties in section 27 of the UIL Constitution and Contest Rules will be applied.

Upon notification that their school has been selected for an anabolic steroid testing event, the MSR will be required to provide an accurate and current list of all student-athletes in grades 9–12 participating in UIL athletic activities at the their school to Drug Free Sport for student-athlete random selection.

The MSR will be required to submit the list within the time frame specified by Drug Free Sport in their notification. The school is required to utilize the UIL Anabolic Steroid Testing Student-Athlete Listing Form, which is available for download on the UIL web site.

The TSCs must select the facilities required for anabolic steroid testing . . .

Day of Anabolic Steroid Testing

Upon arrival at the selected school, the anabolic steroid testing crew chief will provide the MSR with a list of the randomly selected student-athletes for anabolic steroid testing. The randomly selected student-athletes will be notified of and scheduled for anabolic steroid testing by the MSR. The MSR, will notify the student-athlete in person to report immediately to the collection station.

The MSR will have the student-athlete read and sign the UIL Student-Athlete Notification Form. The time of notification will be recorded on the form. The student-athlete will report for anabolic steroid testing immediately upon notification. Student athletes should be reminded to bring photo identification (if available) to the test site.

The MSR will schedule the appropriate number of student athletes to report to anabolic steroid testing as agreed upon by the crew chief and MSR to allow for proper room control. All student-athletes should not be scheduled to arrive at the same time.

UIL member school personnel will be present in the collection station at all times to certify the identity of student-athletes who cannot provide photo identification and will be responsible for security of the collection station at all times.

Only those persons authorized by the crew chief or the UIL member school TSCs will be allowed in the collection station.

Should there be disagreement over who is allowed in the collection station, the decision of the crew chief will prevail.

The TSCs may provide fluids for student-athletes during the anabolic steroid test if necessary . . .

Student-athletes should be warned that over-hydrating will increase the time they spend in anabolic steroid testing. The crew tests the specific gravity of the specimen and dilute specimens will delay the process. No more than three alkaline specimens will be collected. The third alkaline specimen will be packaged and sent to the Laboratory.

Testing Crews
Anabolic Steroid Testing Collection Crews

Drug Free Sport provides the collection crews for each UIL anabolic steroid testing event.

Collection crews are comprised of a crew chief and testing crew members that assist the crew chief. Testing crews could consist of a crew chief, collector, monitor and processing collector. Members of the crew can, and often do, perform multiple roles within the testing crew.

Crew chiefs are trained and certified sport urine specimen collectors. Each crew chief is responsible for training the collection crew.

No member of an anabolic steroid testing crew may participate in anabolic steroid testing at a UIL member high school at which they are employed, or at which they would have any other conflict of interest as determined by the UIL.

The crew chief will make travel and lodging arrangements for his/her crew. Crews will provide their own transportation.

Transportation of specimens to the laboratory and any supplies to Drug Free Sport are the responsibility of the crew chief.

UIL Member School and Student-Athlete Selection

The method for randomly selecting UIL member high schools or student-athletes to be tested for anabolic steroids will be approved by the UIL in advance of the anabolic steroid testing event, administered by Drug Free Sport and implemented by the assigned anabolic steroid testing crew chief.

Student-athletes in the 9th, 10th, 11th and 12th grades at UIL member high schools are subject to random selection for anabolic steroid testing.

Student-athletes will be randomly selected from the official list of all student-athletes in grades 9–12 participating in UIL athletic activities provided by the MSR. The school is required to utilize the UIL Anabolic Steroid Testing Student-Athlete Listing Form, which is available for download on the UIL web site.

A substitute, who will also have been randomly selected, will be made for a student-athlete who is selected for anabolic steroid testing but is absent from school on the day of anabolic steroid testing. Randomly selected student-athletes who do not appear for testing for reasons other than an excused absence will be treated as if there was a positive test result for an anabolic steroid and subject to applicable penalties.

UIL Anabolic Steroid List

- androstenediol
- androstenedione
- boldenone
- chlorotestosterone (4-chlortestosterone)
- clostebol
- dehydrochlormethyltestosterone
- dehydroepiandrosterone (DHEA)
- dihydrotestosterone (DHT)
- dromostanolone
- drostanolone
- epitrenbolone
- ethylestrenol
- fluoxymesterone
- formebulone
- gestrinone
- mesterolone
- methandienone
- methandranone
- methandrostenolone
- methenolone
- methyltestosterone
- mibolerone
- methandriol
- nandrolone
- norandrostenediol
- norandrostenedione
- norethandrolone
- oxandrolone
- oxymesterone
- oxymetholone
- stanolone
- stanozolol
- testolactone
- testosterone*
- tetrahydrogestrinone (THG)
- trenbolone
- and any substance, such as a compound or metabolite, that is chemically or pharmacologically related to testosterone, other than an estrogen, progestin, or corticosteroid, and promotes muscle growth

* For testosterone the definition of positive depends on an adverse analytical finding (positive result) based on the methods listed in section 1.2, which shows that the testosterone is of exogenous origin, or if the ratio of the total concentration of testosterone to that of epitestosterone in the urine is greater than 6:1, unless there is evidence that this ratio is due to a physiological or pathological condition. Student-athletes who provide a urine specimen with a T/E of greater than 6:1 may be subject to additional tests to determine if the T/E ratio is elevated due to exogenous use of testosterone or due to a physiological or pathological condition.

TIMELINE FOR STEROID-RELATED ISSUES (ANABOLIC AND CATABOLIC)

1546	Girolamo Fracastoro reintroduced the germ theory to the modern era.
1676	Antonie van Leenwenhock discovered microorganisms using microscope, also discovered red blood cells and spermatozoa.
1815	Eugène Charreul identifies cholesterine as a form of bile.
1833	M. F. Boudet identifies cholesterine in the blood.
1854	John Snow uses microscope to an isolated cause of cholera outbreak.
1860	August Wilhelm von Hafman uses three-dimensional models to illustrate molecular structure, giving birth to stereochemistry.
1865	Amsterdam swimmers charged with taking dope.
1869	Cyclists caught using speedballs (a combination of heroin and cocaine).
1874	Jacob Henricus van't Hoff earned the first Nobel Prize for chemistry.
1878	Wilhelm Kühre discovered enzymes.
1894	Pierre de Coubertin organizes first International Olympic Committee.
1890	The word cholesterol coined to describe cholesterine after it was identified as an alcohol.
1891	Active ingredient responsible for hallucinogenic properties of mescaline identified by Arthur Heffter.
1893	Nagai Nogayoshi first synthesizes methamphetamine from ephedrine.
1896	Cycling coach/manager, James "Choppy" Warburton banned by Britain's National Cycling Union for allegations that he routinely doped his athletes.
1903	English Jockey Club banned doping of horses and developed a saliva test for cocaine and heroin in 1910.
1904	U.S. marathoner Thomas Hicks collapses after ingesting a brew of strychnine and brandy to win the Olympic race.

1905   The word hormone first coined by Ernest Starling to describe chemical messengers that pass from cell to cell to enable metabolic function.

1912   Friedrich Gudernatsch discovers certain hormones could be active across species.

1919   Akira Ogata synthesizes a crystal form of methamphetamine also known as speed.

1920   Carl Mannich synthesizes hydrocodone as an opioid derived from codeine.

1923   X-Ray Diffraction used to identify fatty acids.

1926   Charles R. Harrington synthesized first hormone, thyroxine.

1926   Fred Koch and Lemuel McGee synthesized testosterone from bull testes.

1927   Adolf Windaus and Heinrich Otto Wieland identify correct structure of cholesterol, and earn Nobel Prize in 1928.

1928   Alexander Fleming first discovers penicillin.

1928   International Amateur Athletic Foundation bans doping of human athletes, but with no testing procedures.

1929   Adolf Butenandt first isolates estrone, and earns Noble Prize in 1939. Edward Doisy also isolated estrone independently in 1930.

1930   International Horse Racing Organization required tests on all horses.

1931   Aldous Huxley published *Brave New World*, in which a future world is dominated by a dictatorship that used drugs to sedate its population into submission.

1931   Electromicroscope invented by Max Knoll and Ernst Ruska, and used to track molecular synthesis.

1932   Smith Kline marketed methamphetamines under name of Benzadrine as an inhaler used to treat blocked sinus passages.

1934   Edward Kendall purifies and isolates cortisone.

1935   Ernest Laqueur isolated molecular structure of male hormone, which he names testosterone.

1935   Adolf Butenandt and Leopold Ruzicka independently synthesized testosterone, and earned Nobel Prize in 1939.

1935   Charles Kochakian defined characteristics of testosterone.

1936   The word steroid first used to describe derivative of cholesterol.

1937   Smith Kline sold methamphetamines in pill form.

1938   Albert Hofmann synthesizes lysergic acid diethylamide (LSD) from ergotamine.

1938   Warren Weaver uses X-ray crystallography to identify arrangement of atoms in a crystalline molecule.

1941   Charles Fletcher first uses penicillin to fight infection.

1943   Hallucinogenic properties of LSD discovered.

1945	Ernst Chevin and Howard Florey discover method for mass production of penicillin.
1945	Olympic runner Gundar Hägg set world record by running the mile in 4 minutes and 1 second.
1949	Philip Hench and Edward Kendall publish research using cortisone to treat rheumatoid arthritis. Hench and Kendall share a Nobel Prize the following year.
1950	Danish Sports Federation informally accused of doping their rowing teams.
1950	Gas Chromatography used to identify molecular characteristics.
1951	Carl Djerassi and others synthesize progestin norethindrone, which will later become the first oral contraceptive.
1951	Methaqualone synthesized in India by Kishore Kacker and Syed Hussein Zaheer.
1952	Bob Hoffman, U.S. Olympic weightlifting team coach, informally accuses Soviet weightlifting team with using some kind of ergogenic drug.
1952	Phencyclidine (also known as PCP) patented and marketed for therapeutic use as an antipsychotic in 1952; it was first synthesized in 1926.
1953	Parke-Davis and Company sued for falsely advertising chloromycetin as completely nontoxic. The drug was linked to death of several children.
1954	American College of Sports Medicine (ACSM) formed.
1954	Bob Hoffman and John Ziegler received confirmation from the Soviet team physician that their weightlifting team was taking testosterone.
1954	Roger Bannister became the first runner to break the four-minute mile barrier, which was repeated by 12 runners on 18 occasions during the three years that followed.
1955	Meprobamate marketed by Wallace Laboratories as a mild antianxiety drug under the name Miltown.
1956	Australian swim team informally accused to doping.
1957	Albert Hofman synthesized active ingredient in psilocybin mushroom to use as an antipsychotic.
1957	hGH developed by Genentech Inc. to treat dwarfism in children.
1957	Thalidomide released by Grünental as a nonbarbiturate sedative, resulting in more than 10,000 cases of phocomela. It was never approved for use in the United States.
1960	Twenty-three-year-old cyclist Knud Jensen dies while racing during the Rome Olympics.
1960	Timothy Leary began testing effect of LSD on rehabilitation of paroled prisoners in what became known as the "Concord Prison Experiment."
1962	President John F. Kennedy signs the Food, Drug and Cosmetic Act, which established stricter consumer protections for pharmaceutical

companies and empowered FDA with authority to track and regulate the development and advertisement of pharmaceuticals in the United States.

1962   Dihydrotestosterone (sold as stanazolol) was approved by the FDA as a therapeutic treatment for hypogonadism.

1963   Dianabol introduced during the San Diego Chargers training camp by Strength Training coach, Alvin Roy.

1963   Ken Kesey tours college campuses promoting LSD as a recreational drug.

1965   Computer program DENDRAL created to illustrate molecular structure from unknown organic compounds.

1965   France and Belgium passes laws banning ergogenic drugs in sports.

1965   IOC sponsors an International Conference on Doping to look into potential anti-doping policies and enforcement methods.

1966   International Cycling Union and International Football Federation ban ergogenic drugs.

1966   U.S. federal congress followed example of most states and bans LSD as a controlled substance.

1967   English cyclist, Tom Simpson, dies during Tour de France.

1967   Steroids developer, John Ziegler, publicly condemns anabolic steroid use for athletes.

1967   IOC defines doping and creates a list of prohibited substances for Olympian athletes, but does not initiate comprehensive testing until 1976.

1967   IOC introduces chromosomal gender tests for winning athletes.

1969   FDA issues advertising guidelines requiring pharmaceutical companies to include complete summaries of risks and benefits associated with each drug in ads targeting consumers directly.

1969   *Sports Illustrated* article "Drugs in Sports" claims that anyone entering professional football since 1965 has used steroids.

1970   President Richard Nixon signs the Controlled Substance Act, creating five schedules to classify drugs according to their risk of addiction and their potential use as a therapeutic treatment.

1972   Bjorn Ekblöm invents a method of packing an athlete's blood oxygen levels through transfusion, resulting in 25 percent improvement in endurance.

1972   Informal poll of Track and Field competitors at the 1972 Olympics indicates 68 percent used steroids to prepare for the games.

1973   IOC introduced radioimmunoassay and gas chromatography tests to detect steroid use among Olympians. First used at the 1976 Olympic Games.

1973   U.S. Senate Subcommittee holds hearings on "Drugs and Athletics."

1974 IOC revises charter to include provisions that establish automatic suspension for athletes refusing to take or failing to pass drug tests.

1975 IOC added steroids to the list of banned substances.

1976 Rich DeMint stripped of Olympic Gold after testing positive for ephedrine. He later appealed on grounds that he used beta-2 bronchospasmolytic to treat his asthma. DeMint did not win his case, but IOC established protocols for therapeutic use exemptions (TUE).

1981 Food, Drug and Cosmetic Act revised requiring prescriptions for anabolic steroids for therapeutic use only. No penalties were included for enforcement.

1981 Merck runs first direct-to-consumer print ad for a prescription medicine (pneumovax) since the FDA gained regulatory authority over advertising guidelines in 1962.

1982 Manfred Donike develops the T/E test for testosterone, which was introduced at the 1983 Pan American games, resulting in 19 positive tests and dozens of competitors leaving early before their events.

1983 The East German Sport program begins using DHT, androstenedione, DHEA, and other precursor supplements to evade the existing T/E testosterone tests used by the IOC.

1984 U.S. Olympic Committee began testing for steroids during Olympic trials; 86 failed the tests. No sanctions were imposed.

1985 hGH extracted from human cadavers linked to Creutzfeldt-Jakob disease, prompting the creation of a synthetic version the same year.

1985 Joint Task Force, including FDA, DEA, U.S. Customs, U.S. Postal Service, and FBI launch investigation of steroid trafficking into the United States. Results in the seizure of 440 cases (worth $16 million) and indictments of 110 individuals in 1987.

1986 IOC bans blood doping.

1987 IOC began requesting that athletes be tested at training camps as well as during competitions.

1988 Canadian runner Ben Johnson and U.S. runner Florence Griffith-Joyner were stripped of their medals after positive drug tests (for hGH and stanozolol) following the 1988 Olympic Games.

1988 President Ronald Reagan signs Anti-Drug Abuse Act, which outlaws sale of anabolic steroids for nontherapeutic purposes.

1990 Anabolic Steroids Control Act reclassifies anabolic steroids for nontherapeutic purposes as a Schedule III controlled substance.

1991 East Germany sports officials admit to long history of organized steroid abuse.

1991 MLB Commissioner Fay Vincent sends out a memo to all teams warning that all illegal drug use is prohibited (which includes anabolic steroids).

1992   American Medical Association (AMA) approves direct-to-consumer pharmaceutical advertising.

1992   IOC establishes reduced T/E from 6:1 to 4:1.

1992   Professional football player, Lyle Alzado, dies of brain cancer. He and his family blamed the cancer on steroid use.

1994   During the Asian games, the Chinese swim team is subjected to surprise drug tests, resulting in 11 athletes testing positive and stripped of 22 medals.

1998   Festina Scandal erupts during the Tour de France race, leading to the formation of WADA as an independent anti-doping agency in 1999.

1999   BALCO sells first synthetic steroid (norbolethone) designed to beat doping tests.

1999   FDA changes advertising guidelines allowing broadcast ads to limit their "fair and balanced" disclosure responsibilities to brief summaries of major risks and a provision for more information elsewhere.

1999   World Anti-Doping Agency (WADA) formed as an independent agency, with funds that come equally from sports movements and national governments.

2000   U.S. Anti-doping Agency (USADA) formed as an independent agency

2002   Norbolethone identified and detected by WADA, bringing new attention to the risk of designer steroids.

2004   FDA allows print ads the freedom to use simplified language and list only a summary of major risks associated with prescription drugs when presented directly to the consumer (the same as broadcast ads).

2004   Senate Commerce Committee holds hearings investigating anabolic steroid use in professional sports.

2004   President George W. Bush signs Anabolic Steroid Control Act, which reclassifies steroid precursors among Schedule III controlled substances.

2012   Marijuana for recreational use legalized for the first time at the state level in Colorado and Washington.

2012   United Kingdom bans the import of anabolic steroids for ergogenic use. Prehormones and designer steroids remain legal for individual use.

Glossary

Abortifacient: Any artificial chemical or device that induces an abortion. Some oral contraceptives work by destroying the ovum after fertilization, thereby inducing a very early abortion.

Acromegaly: A disease that results in excessive growth in flat bones, especially the lower jaw, hands, and feet, as well as certain soft tissues on the face and in abdominal organs (sometimes called gigantism). A known side effect of excessive hGH.

Addison's disease: A potentially terminal wasting disease characterized by muscle weakness, drowsiness, weight loss, and other skin and gastrointestinal disturbances. Caused by disordered adrenal glands. *See also* Aldosterone.

Adenosine triphosphate (ATP): The source of energy used by muscles to build and repair tissues. Occurs naturally in the body, but may also be stimulated by outside supplements. *See also* Creatine.

Aldosterone: A mineralocorticoid steroid hormone synthesized in the adrenal cortex and sent to the kidneys, where it is largely responsible for regulating electrolyte levels, blood pressure, and volume. *See also* Renin-angiotensin-aldosterone cascade.

Alternative medicine: Any system of healing that is not included in the traditional curriculum of medical schools in Europe and the United States, because it assumes healing opportunities outside the norms of clinical research.

Amphetamine: A chemical compound used to stimulate the central nervous system. Ergogenic use is banned by anti-doping policies of almost all sports associations. *See also* Ephedrine and Methamphetamine.

Anabolism: Metabolic operations help to construct compounds at the molecular level. A major function of anabolic steroids used to help repair and build tissues in the human body. *See also* Metabolism and Catabolism.

Analogue (chemical): A compound that closely resembles the structure and function of another chemical. Typically used by pharmaceutical companies when the original composing is not easily accessible or may include less desirable characteristics.

Androgens: Hormones used in male reproduction. *See also* Testosterone.

Androstanes: A class of steroid hormone with only 19 carbon atoms, which includes androgenic steroids.

Androstenedione: The chemical source for both testosterone and estrone, which is synthesized in the adrenal cortex and sex organs. *See also* Dianabol.

Anovulent: Any chemical compound used to prevent ovulation. Initially developed as an oral contraceptive.

Anthranilic acid: A class of cholestanes derived from benzoic acid, from which tryptophan amino acids are synthesized. Also known as vitamin L, which is an essential part of the human diet. *See also* Cholestanes and Benzoic acid.

Autologous blood doping: When athletes transfuse their own stored oxygenated blood to improve endurance and performance. *See also* Blood doping and Homologous blood doping.

BALCO: Acronym for the pharmaceutical company called the Bay Area Laboratory Co-Operative, which specialized in synthesis of ergogenic drugs. BALCO became the center of a steroids scandal in 2003, which implicated dozens of professional athletes, and eventually led to congressional hearings to investigate the prevalence of steroids in professional sports. *See also* Designer steroid.

Benzoic acid: A class of cholestanes that was used as a food preserver from as early as the 16th century. Used today by pharmaceutical companies as a reagent and to extend the shelf life of drugs. *See also* Cholestanes and Anthranilic acid.

Blood doping: A procedure developed by a Swedish researcher to improve endurance and performance of elite athletes by transfusing the highly oxygenated blood prior to competition. The added red blood cells increases the amount of oxygen carried to the muscles. Blood doping was banned by the IOC in 1986, though no tests were available to detect autologous blood doping until 2012. *See also* Homologous blood doping and Autologous blood doping.

Catabolism: Metabolic operations help to break down compounds at the molecular level. A major function of catabolic steroids is to release energy and disassemble complex molecules. *See also* Metabolism and Anabolism.

Cell membranes: The semipermeable layer composed of cholesterol surrounding cell protoplasm in human physiology. In plant biology, the layer surrounding a cell is called a cell wall in plant cells.

Cholagogue: Any chemical compound that increases the production and flow of bile.

Cholane: A class of nonsteroid hormones, also known as cholic acids.

Choleretic: A property of cholane hormones, which stimulates the production and flow of bile in the liver and the gall bladder. *See also* Cholagogue and Cholane.

Cholestanes: A class of nonhormone steroids composed of 27 carbons, with two methyl substituents attached to the 17th carbon atom. Derivatives include glycosides, saponins, benzoic acids, secosteroids, and sterols. *See also* Cholesterol.

Cholesterol: A nonhormone steroid used as precursor for almost all steroid hormones, and controls the fluidity of cell membranes.

The Code: The specific list of prohibited ergogenic drugs, devices, and procedures identified by WADA, and serves as the model for most other anti-doping policies worldwide.

Corticosteroids: The catabolic half of steroids in the pregnane molecular group that are most responsible for regulating metabolism, immunity, and also influencing memory functions. *See also* Pregnane.

Cortisol: A glucocorticoid steroid that enhances the expression of enzymes to facilitate the formation of glucose in the liver. Cortisol is essential for proper brain functioning, including memory, learning, and mood. *See also* Gluconeogenesis.

Creatine: A chemical produced naturally in muscle tissues, which increases ATP levels providing muscles with more energy to build and repair themselves. Synthetic versions may be taken as a dietary supplement and is legal without a prescription. Side effects include fluid retention and may interfere with kidney function.

Creutzfeldt-Jakob disease: A fatal neurological disease that gradually degrades brain tissues leading to early dementia and loss of muscle coordination. *See also* hGH.

Cushing's syndrome: A disease resulting from too much cortisol, which is characterized by fat deposits in the neck, trunk, and face; thinning of the skin leading to bruises; high blood pressure; and other emotional effects. *See also* Cortisol.

Cycling: Term used to describe a technique of taking multiple doses of anabolic steroids for a sustained period of time, stopping for a period of rest, and then resuming the process. Users cycle steroids in an attempt to limit the cumulative side effects. *See also* Stacking and Pyramiding.

Dehydroepiandrosterone (DHEA): A precursor to both testosterone and estradiol, which is naturally synthesized in the body from pregnenolone and which is used to create both testosterone and estradiol. Marketed as an antiaging supplement and sold legally in the United States as a dietary supplement, though prohibited by WADA and most anti-doping policies.

Designer steroid: Any steroid synthesized for the specific purpose of evading existing anti-doping policies. The first designer steroid was developed by BALCO. *See also* BALCO.

Dianabol: The first synthetic testosterone analogue marketed in the United States. *See also* Androstenedione.

Dihydrotestosterene (DHT): The primary male sex hormone derived from testosterone, which is responsible for building muscles as well as other male characteristics such as facial and body hair growth and deeper voice. An anabolic steroid prohibited by WADA and other anti-doping policies when used for ergogenic effect.

Direct-to-consumer (marking): The practice of advertising pharmaceuticals directly to the patient through radio, television, internet, and print media. An alternative to advertising indirectly through the advice of a physician.

Dope: The term used to describe any substance used to influence the performance of an athlete (animal or human) during competition.

Drug lag: The time it takes between when a drug treatment is discovered and when it can be made legally available to the public.

Endocrine system: The complex of functions that coordinates the production or inhibition of chemical compounds used to regulate most of our metabolic functions. *See also* Hormones.

Enzyme-linked immunosorbent assay (ELISA): A simple testing method used to detect prohibited substances in racing animals.

Ephedrine: An adrenaline analogue used to stimulate the central nervous system. Ergogenic use is banned by anti-doping policies of almost all sports associations. *See also* Amphetamine and Methamphetamine.

EPO: A glycoprotein hormone marketed under the name of Epogen, which was approved by the FDA as a treatment for anemia. Used by athletes as a synthetic form of blood doping. Prohibited by WADA as an ergogenic drug. *See also* Blood doping.

Ergogenic: Any method, chemical or physical device, used to enhance performance.

Estradiol: A female sex hormone derived from pregnenolone and secreted through follicles in the ovaries. After ovulation, the same cells produce progesterone, which is used to prepare the uterus for implantation of the ovum.

Estranes: A class of anabolic steroids hormone with 18 carbons, which includes female sex hormones. *See also* Estradiol, Estrogens, and Progestogins.

Estrogens: The term used to categorize the female steroids. *See also* Estrone, Estradiol, and Progestogins.

Estrone: The female sex steroid synthesized in the ovaries, and most responsible for sexual reproduction and secondary sex characteristics of women. *See also* Estrogens.

Eunuch: Any male who has lost the use of the testes.

Feedback loops: The term used to describe hormone reaction chains within the endrocrine system that guards against overproduction or underproduction of hormones and enzymes that govern most metabolic activity.

Festina scandal: A series of doping-related incident during the 1998 Tour de France, which seemed to confirm the existence of coordinated evasion among teams from Western Democracies.

Genes: The DNA strands that determine the particular characteristics of the organism, and which are responsible for the synthesis of certain proteins.

Glucocorticoid: A class of catabolic hormones synthesized by the adrenal glands, which are responsible for regulating the amount of sugar (mostly glucose) in the body.

Gluconeogenesis: The process of forming glucose in the liver, mostly triggered by the cortisol steroid. *See also* Cortisol.

Glycolysis: The process of breaking glucose down into its intermediate parts resulting in releasing energy that is then stored in the ATP. *See also* Adenosine triphosphate (ATP).

Glycosides: A class of nonhormonal steroid that is chemically derived from cholestanes with 27 carbon atoms. They affect hormone-producing tissues and produce yields that separate sugars and nonsugars. It is the main ingredient in digitalus.

Gonane: The name of the core chemical structure shared by all steroid, which includes 17 carbon atoms arranged in three cyclohexane (six-membered) rings and one cyclopentane (five-membered) ring connected side by side.

HDL: High-density lipoproteins often referred to as good cholesterol because they can collect the low-density lipoprotein (LDL) packets and clean out artery pathways. *See also* LDL and Lipoproteins.

Hermaphroditism: A biological disorder that occurs when an individual possesses both male and female reproductive organs (though usually not in equal proportions).

hGH: Human growth hormones. A polypeptide hormone is synthesized by the pituitary gland, and is responsible for new cell production and bone growth. The hormone converts insulin into a growth factor for bones, muscles, and other tissues.

Homeostasis: The state of harmonious balance of hormones and enzymes in the endocrine system.

Homologous blood doping: When highly oxygenated blood from another person is transfused into an athlete prior to competition to improve endurance and performance. *See also* Blood doping and Autologous blood doping.

Hormones: Specialized chemical compounds that affect the permeability of cell membranes, govern the rate of chemical reactions (including cascading chains of reactions), activate or inhibit enzyme systems, and influence the functions of genes at the chromosomal level.

Hydrophobic: The characteristics of certain molecules that do not dissolve or mix with water. Steroid hormones are fat soluble and hydrophobic.

Hypertension: A condition of abnormally high blood pressure. *See also* Aldosterone.

In vitro: The process of chemical synthesis that occurs in a laboratory. *See also* In vivo.

In vivo: The process of chemical synthesis that occurs through the metabolic function of another living organism. *See also* In vitro.

LDL: Low-density lipoprotein packets, often called bad cholesterol, tend to build up on the internal walls of the blood vessels and can potentially create a buildup in the arteries leading to heart disease. *See also* HDL and Lipoproteins.

Leukocytes: White blood cells produced from white bone marrow used by the body to defend and neutralize foreign substances, often resulting in localized inflammation.

Leydig cells: Cells within the testes that convert cholesterol into pregnenolone, then to androstenedione, and then to testosterone. *See also* Dihydrotestosterene and Estradiol.

Lipoproteins: The protein-covered packets of cholesterol used to send messages from one system to the next, and which trigger various feedback loops. *See also* LDL and HDL.

Lysergic acid diethylamide (LSD): Commonly known as acid. A compound derived from ergotamine, which produces hallucinogenic properties. Originally created as an antipsychotic therapy, it later became a recreational drug during the 1960s. *See also* Psychedelic drugs.

Metabolism: The broad processes of biochemical reactions needed to sustain all life, including both the construction and destruction of tissues in a living body. *See also* Anabolism and Catabolism.

Methamphetamine: A chemical compound used to stimulate the central nervous system, banned by almost all sports associations; first discovered in Japan during the 1880s. *See also* Amphetamine.

Methandrostenalone: A synthetic version of androstenedione developed by John Ziegler as the first commercially available anabolic steroid. *See also* Androstenedione and Dianabol.

Mineralocorticoids: A class of catabolic steroids that regulates inorganic materials such as sodium and potassium and produced in the adrenal cortex.

Moiety: A chemical term meaning part that refers to the substituent chain that extends off the steroid gonane to distinguish one steroid from another. *See also* Substituent and Gonane.

mRNA: Abbreviation of messenger ribonucleic acid, which acts in a cell's nucleus and copies relevant strands on the DNA chain to activate (or inhibit) whatever operation that cell was programmed to undertake. *See also* Transcription and Ribosomes.

Norethindrone: The first analogue synthesis of progesterone, a progestogin that acts as an oral contraceptive. *See also* Progestogins.

Placebo effect: The phenomenon that occurs when people believe that the treatment they are taking will produce the desired results.

Prader-Willi syndrome: A disorder resulting in small genitalia, mental retardation, and obesity. Treatments include hGH. *See also* hGH.

Prednisone: A synthetic form of cortisol commercially available since the 1950s, and used as an anti-inflammatory. *See also* Cortisol.

Pregnanes: A class of hormone steroids with 21 carbons, derived from cholesterol.

Progestogins: Sex-related (anabolic) hormones that are mostly responsible for female reproduction. They share the same 21 carbon skeletal structure as the catabolic mineralocorticoids and glucocorticoids. *See also* Estrone, Estradiol, and Norethindrone.

Psychedelic drugs: A popular classification of drugs that produce hallucinogenic effects. *See also* Lysergic acid diethylamide (LSD).

Pyramiding: The practice of gradually escalating the dose and frequency of a steroid to reach a peak at mid-cycle before gradually tapering down toward the end of the cycle. *See also* Cycling and Stacking.

Rational design: Creating specific molecules to control substrates or receptors for particular enzymes, hormones, and neurotransmitters.

Rennin-angiotensin-aldosterone cascade: A complex feedback system that regulates electrolyte levels, blood pressure, and volume. *See also* Aldosterone.

Ribosomes: An acid molecule that interacts with mRNA and links amino acids together to create particular proteins. *See also* mRNA and Transcription.

Rickets: A disease that causes bone and cartilage tissues to fail in higher life forms, and treatable with vitamin D. *See also* Vitamin D.

Saponins: A type of glycosides characterized by their foaming reaction and used in soap. *See also* Glycosides.

Schedules (controlled substances): The classification system by which controlled substances is listed according to their recognized potential for abuse; accepted therapeutic value for medical use; and relative safety under medical supervision.

Scientific method: A formal system for identifying, evaluating, and testing new knowledge.

Secondary sex traits: The physical characteristics that most distinguish men and women.

Secosteroids: A category of nonhormone steroids with a cholestane chemical structure, also known as vitamin D. *See also* Cholestane and Vitamin D.

Sex steroids: The anabolic steroid hormones responsible for reproduction and tissue growth, including progestogins, andrane, and estrane molecular groups. *See also* Progestogins and Testosterone.

Stacking: The practice of taking multiple steroids simultaneously.

Stereochemistry: The study of the physical structure of atoms to understand chemical properties.

Steroidogenesis: The synthesis of steroids within the body.

Sterols: A category of cholestanes found in the tissues of virtually all life forms—plant and animal (with the exception of some forms of algae and bacteria). *See also* Cholestanes.

Substituent: A moiety that substitutes the hydrogen atom on the steroid gonane with part of another molecule.

Synthesis pathway: The steps by which a chemical is synthesized in a laboratory setting.

Synthetic hormones: Analogue versions of natural hormones. *See also* Analogue (chemical).

Systemic reaction: Any physiological change that affects the entire body.

T/E ratio: The ratio between glucuroconjugated testosterone to epitestosterone used to test for the presence of testosterone introduced from outside the body, and is a significant tool for anti-doping enforcement worldwide.

Testosterone: The key anabolic steroid responsible for male sex characteristics.

Thalidomide: A nonbarbiturate-based sedative responsible for thousands of birth defects worldwide. Led to the Food, Drug and Cosmetic Act of 1962.

THC: Abbreviation for delta-9-tetrahydrocannabinol, which is the active ingredient of marijuana.

Therapeutic use exemptions (TUE): Specific exceptions identified by WADA for medically prescribed (therapeutic) use of anabolic steroids or other drugs with potential ergogenic effects.

Thresholds (testing): The method used by anti-doping officials to distinguish between drugs administered by a certified veterinarian for therapeutic purposes and those used for ergogenic purposes in animals.

Tracer techniques: A method for tracking the changes in molecular structure after synthesis.

Transcription: The process of copying a DNA strand to produce the mRNA necessary to inhibit or activate a function of a particular cell. *See also* mRNA, Ribosomes, and Translation (chemical).

Translation (chemical): The entire process by which a molecule activates (or inhibits) the operation that a cell was programmed to undertake. Also referred to as the expression of a gene's function. *See also* mRNA, Ribosomes, and Transcription.

USADA: The U.S. Anti-Doping Agency (USADA), which is an independent body responsible for ensuring the integrity and commitment of amateur sports associations.

Vitamin D: A nonhormone steroid used for the metabolism of calcium, which helps to strengthen bone tissues. *See also* Secosteroids.

Vitamins: Any substance that is essential to human metabolism, not naturally synthesized by the human body, and which can only be extracted from certain foods.

Whey proteins: A dietary supplement containing nutrients from the watery portion of milk extracted from curds during the process of making cheese. Used to promote muscle growth and may include natural anti-inflammatory properties, but is not prohibited by WADA.

Zero tolerance: A policy that means even trace amounts will result in a failed doping test.

FURTHER READING

Amerson, Katherine. *Direct-to-Consumer Pharmaceutical Advertising in Men's and Women's Magazines*, M.A. Thesis. Lubbock: Texas Tech University, 2007.

Assael, Shaun. *Steroid Nation: Juiced Home Run Totals, Anti-Aging Miracles, and a Hercules in Every High-school—The Secret History of America's True Drug Addiction*. New York: ESPN, 2007.

Ayotte, Christiane. "Detecting the Administration of Endogenous Anabolic Androgenic Steroids." In *Handbook of Experimental Pharmacology*, edited by Walter Rosenthal, 77–98. Quebec, Canada: Springer, 2010.

Bahrke, Michael S., and Charles Yesalis, eds. *Performance-Enhancing Substances in Sport and Exercise*. Champaign, IL: Human Kinetics, 2002.

Barber D, P. Ghorbani, and O. Wenker. "Supplemental Steroids in the Operating Room: A review of the Literature." *Internet Journal of Anesthesiology* 1, no. 1(1997), http://www.ispub.com/journals/IJA/Vol1N1/articles/steroid.htm.

Beamish, Rob. *Steroids: A New Look at Performance-Enhancing Drugs*. Santa Barbara, CA: Praeger, 2011.

Bernard, Robert W. *Secret of Rejuvenation: Professor Brown Sequard's Great Discovery of the Fountain of Youth*. London: Society of Metaphysicians, 1999 [c.1956].

Berryman, Jack W., and Roberta J. Park, eds. *Sport and Exercise Science: Essays in the History of Sports Medicine*. Chicago: University of Illinois Press, 1992.

Black, Lee. "Limiting Parents' Rights in Medical Decision Making." *Virtual Mentor: American Medical Association Journal of Ethics* 8, no. 10(2006): 676–80.

Bryant, Howard. *Juicing the Game: Drugs, Power, and the Fight for the Soul of Major League Baseball*. New York: Viking Press, 2005.

Burge, John. "Legalize and Regulate: A Prescription for Reforming Anabolic Steroid Legislation." *Loyola of Los Angeles Entertainment Law Review* 15, no. 33(1994): 33–60.

Burns, Christopher, ed. *Doping in Sports*. New York: Nova Science Publishers, 2006.

Dimeo, Paul. *A History of Drug Use in Sport 1876–1976*. New York: Routledge, 2007.

Djerassi, Carl. *Steroids Made It Possible*. Washington, DC: American Chemical Society, 1990.

Fainaru-Wada, Mark, and Lance Williams. *Game of Shadows: Barry Bonds, BALCO, and the Steroids Scandal that Rocked Professional Sports*. New York: Gotham Books, 2007.

Gandert, Daniel, and Fabian Ronisky. "American Professional Sports is a Doper's Paradise: It's Time We Make a Change." *North Dakota Law Review–Sports Law Symposium* 86, no. 4(2010): 813–44.

Gerdes, Louise, ed. *At Issue: Performance Enhancing Drugs*. New York: Greenhaven Press, 2008.

Gober, Sarita, Malky Klein, Tzippy Berger, Cristina Vindigni, and Paul C. McCabe. "Steroids in Adolescence: The Cost of Achieving a Physical Ideal." *NASP Communiqué* 37, no. 7(2006): 132–32.

Goldman, Bob, Patricia Bush, and Ronald Klatz. *Death in the Locker Room: Steroids, Cocaine & Sports*. Tucson, AZ: The Body Press, 1984.

Hamilton, Tyler, and Daniel Coyle. *The Secret Race: Inside the Hidden World of the Tour de France—Doping, Cover-ups, and Winning at All Costs*. New York: Bantam, 2012.

Hansen, J. R. *Introduction to Steroid Chemistry*. New York: Pergamon Press, 1968.

Heftmann, Erich, and Erich Mosettig. *Biochemistry of Steroids*. New York: Reinhold Publishing Corporation, 1960.

Herzberg, David. *Happy Pills in America: From Miltown to Prozac*. Baltimore, MD: John Hopkins University Press, 2010.

Hoffman, Jay R., and Nicholas Ratamess. "Medical Issues Associated with Anabolic Steroid Use: Are They Exaggerated?" *Journal of Sports Science and Medicine* 5, (2006): 182–93.

Humphrey, Kim R., Kathleen P. Decker, Linn Goldberg, Harrison G. Pope, Joseph Gutman, and Gary Green. "Anabolic Steroid Use and Abuse by Police Officers: Policy & Prevention." *The Police Chief* 75, no. 6(2008): 66–70.

Jayne, Walter Addison. *The Healing Gods of Ancient Civilizations*. Whitefish, MT: Kessinger Publishing, 2010 [c.1925].

Jendrick, Nathan. *Dunks, Doubles, Doping: How Steroids Are Killing American Athletics*. Guilford, CT: The Lyons Press, 2006.

Kim, James H., and Anthony R. Scialli. "Thalidomide: The Tragedy of Birth defects and the Effective Treatment of Disease." *Toxicological Sciences* 122, no. 1(2011): 1–6.

Kochakian, Charles D., ed. *Anabolic-Androgenic Steroids*. New York: Springer-Verlag, 1976.

Kruif, Paul de. *The Male Hormone*. New York: Harcourt, Brace and Company, 1945.

Lenahan, Pat. *Anabolic Steroids and Other Performance-Enhancing Drugs*. New York: Taylor & Francis, 2003.

Lin, Geraline C., and Lynda Erinoff. *Anabolic Steroid Abuse*. Rockville, MD: National Institute on Drug Abuse, 1990.

McCloskey, John, and Julian Bailes. *When Winning Costs Too Much: Steroids, Supplements, and Scandal in Today's Sports*. Lanham, MD: Taylor Trade Publishing, 2005.

Monaghan, Lee F. *Bodybuilding, Drugs and Risk*. New York: Routledge, 2001.

Pearl, Bill. *Getting Stronger: Weight Training for Men & Women*. Rev. ed. Bolinas, CA: Shelter Publications, 2001.

Radomski, Kirk. *Bases Loaded: The Inside Story of the Steroid Era in Baseball by the Central Figure in the Mitchell Report*. New York: Hudson Street Press, 2009.

Rogers, Peter D., and Brian H. Hardin. *Pediatric Clinics of North America: Performance Enhancing Drugs*. Philadelphia: Saunders, 2007.

Rosen, Daniel M. *Dope: A History of Performance Enhancement in Sports from the Nineteenth Century to Today*. Westport, CT: Praeger Publishers, 2008.

Rothman, Sheila, and David Rothman. *The Pursuit of Perfection: The Promise and Perils of Medical Enhancement*. New York: Pantheon Books, 2003.

Tata, Jamshed R. "One Hundred Years of Hormones." *EMBO Reports* 6, no. 6(2005): 490–96.

Taylor, William N. *Anabolic Therapy in Modern Medicine*. Jefferson, NC: McFarland & Company Inc., Publishers, 2002.

Taylor, William N. *Macho Medicine: A History of the Anabolic Steroid Epidemic* Jefferson, NC: McFarland & Company Inc., Publishers, 1991.

Thevis, Mario. *Mass Spectrometry in Sports Drug Testing: Characterization of Prohibited Substances and Doping Control Analytical Assays*. New York: Wiley Publishers, 2010.

Thompson, Teri, Nathaniel Vinton, Michael O'Keefe, and Christian Red. *American Icon: The Fall of Roger Clemens and the Rise of Steroids in America's Pastime*. New York: Alfred A. Knoff, 2009.

Thorne, Gerard. *Anabolic Primer: Ergogenic Enhancement for the Hardcore Bodybuilder*. New York: Robert Kennedy Publishing, 2009.

Tobbell, Dominique A. *Pills, Power, and Policy: The Struggle for Drug Reform in Cold War America and its Consequences*. Berkeley: University of California Press, 2011.

Tone, Andrea. *The Age of Anxiety: A History of America's Turbulent Affair with Tranquilizers*. New York: Basic Books, 2008.

Tricker, Ray, and David L. Cook. *Athletes at Risk: Drugs and Sport*. Dubuque, IA: Wm. C. Brown Publishers, 1990.

United States Congress House of Representatives. *Restoring Faith in America's Pastime: Evaluating Major League Baseball's Efforts to Eradicate Steroid Use*. Washington, DC: BiblioGov, 2010.

Ventola, C. Lee. "Direct-to-Consumer Pharmaceutical Advertising: Therapeutic or Toxic?" *Pharmacy and Therapeutics* 36, no. 10(2011): 669–74, 681–48.

Wadler, Gary, and Brian Hainline. *Drugs and the Athlete: Contemporary Exercise and Sports Medicine*. Philadelphia: F.A. Davis Company, 1989.

Wilson, Wayne, and Edward Derse, eds. *Doping in Elite Sport: The Politics of Drugs in the Olympic Movement*. Champaign, IL: Human Kinetics, 2001.

Yesalis, Charles, and Virginia S. Cowart. *The Steroids Game: An Expert's Inside Look at Anabolic Steroid Use in Sports*. Champaign, IL: Human Kinetics Publishers, 1998.

Yesalis, Charles, ed. *Anabolic Steroids in Sport and Exercise*. Champaign, IL: Human Kinetics Publishers, 1993.

INDEX

ABOUT THE AUTHOR

Aharon W. Zorea, PhD, is a professor at the University of Wisconsin, UW-Richland campus, where he has taught since 2004. He also currently serves as curator for the Wisconsin Historical Society and is the director of the Richland Heritage Project, an independent institute specializing in collecting and digitizing local oral history records, which he founded in 2006. He has written more than 50 articles on 20th-century American policy and culture, including two books—*In the Image of God: A Christian Response to Capital Punishment* and the ABC-CLIO published *Birth Control (Health and Medical Issues Today)*.